Acquiring and Enhancing Physicians' Practices

Steven Portnoy, Ross E. Stromberg, and Philip A. Newbold

In cooperation with the Society for Healthcare Planning and Marketing of the American Hospital Association

American Hospital Publishing, Inc., a wholly owned subsidiary of the American Hospital Association

The views expressed in this book are those of the authors.

Library of Congress Cataloging-in-Publication Data

Portnoy, Steven.
    Acquiring and enhancing physicians' practices

    Includes index.
    1. Hospitals—Business management. 2. Medicine—Practice. I.
Stromberg, Ross E., 1940- . II. Newbold, Philip A. III. Society for
Hospital Planning and Marketing (U.S.). IV. Title. [DNLM: 1. Hospital
Administration. 2. Marketing of Health Services. 3. Practice Management,
Medical. WX 150 P853a]
RA971.3.P67   1988   362.1'1'068   88-19339
ISBN 1-556480-024-5

Catalog no. 145101

Text set in English Times
3M—8/88—0215

Audrey Kaufman, Project Editor
Marcia Bottoms, Managing Editor
Peggy DuMais, Production Coordinator
Marcia Vecchione, Designer
Brian W. Schenk, Books Division Director

Contents

About the Authors

Steven Portnoy is president of Amicus, Inc., a health care consulting firm in Radnor, Pennsylvania, that specializes in market development, strategic planning, and new venture implementation for hospitals, physicians, and other health care providers throughout the country. Mr. Portnoy has been called upon by clients to assist them in the evaluation and implementation of practice acquisition strategies. Before founding Amicus in 1980, Mr. Portnoy served in numerous executive positions as a senior hospital manager and planner, and he has been a manager for health planning and delivery systems for the American Hospital Association. He received a law degree from the Boston University School of Law and is a frequent author and lecturer on the subject of practice acquisition and other aspects of strategic market development.

Ross E. Stromberg is managing partner of the San Francisco office of the law firm Epstein Becker Stromberg & Green. Mr. Stromberg has dedicated his practice to health and hospital law and represents numerous hospitals, multihospital systems, physicians and physician groups, health maintenance organizations, preferred provider organizations, and other forms of managed care delivery systems. Mr. Stromberg is a charter member and past president of the American Academy of Hospital Attorneys of the American Hospital Association. He is a frequent author and lecturer on hospital and health law matters, particularly in the areas of practice acquisition, multi-institutional system development, alternative delivery systems, economic joint venturing, and diversification. Mr. Stromberg is a coauthor of *Joint Ventures for Hospitals and Physicians: Legal Considerations,* published in 1986 by American Hospital Publishing, Inc. He received a law degree from the University of California, Berkeley (the Boalt Hall School of Law).

Philip A. Newbold is president and chief executive officer of Memorial Health Systems, Inc., and Memorial Hospital of South Bend in South Bend, Indiana. Mr. Newbold is a frequent author and lecturer on issues of health care management, marketing, and diversification strategies. He is the founder and former editor of *The Hospital Entrepreneur's Newsletter,* published by Aspen Publishers, Inc. Mr. Newbold has been the recipient of several awards for his innovative leadership in health care administration and marketing. He also lends his considerable leadership talents to various community and civic organizations, and he is past president of the Western Oklahoma Chapter of the Muscular Dystrophy Association. Mr. Newbold received a master of science degree in hospital and health services administration from Ohio State University and a master of business administration degree from Miami University in Oxford, Ohio.

List of Figures

Preface

Have you ever been white-water rafting? For those of us who have not, this appears to be an activity where our risk is great and our control minimal, our triumphs exhilarating and our failures potentially devastating. Such are the views of many hospitals — and, even more so, of many physicians — with respect to practice acquisition.

But those who have experienced the sport can tell you something more. They will tell you that great fulfillment and success are achievable and that survival hinges on many factors — sometimes insight, sometimes the exercise of substantial control, sometimes the relinquishing of control, but always the knowledge of when to use which strategy and the ability to make timely decisions and to adapt to an ever-changing environment. The same is true for the hospital acquiring a physician's practice.

As experienced practitioners in the realm of practice acquisition, the authors offer themselves as your guides through these previously uncharted waters to show you how to use the currents of our changing industry to your best advantage, how to get your team members paddling in the same direction, how to anticipate and avoid the rocks that can threaten your success, and even how and when to bail out when an acquisition vehicle springs a leak too big to repair.

This book was undertaken as a tool for hospital executives seeking practical and specific guidance for considering practice acquisition as a marketing option, for planning for that option, and for implementing the activities critical to the success of the practice acquisition effort. But this is also a book for physicians — from the medical staff leader who is involved on the hospital side to the physician considering the sale of his or her practice to a hospital.

The value of this book should not begin and end with practice acquisition. Such an enterprise is one of many key strategies that fit into the broader scope of physician marketing and practice enhancement. The insights, legal precautions, and practical advice contained herein are relevant for anyone considering the many and varied initiatives that hospitals and physicians can undertake together for their mutual benefit.

We hope that you will regard this book as a kind of life jacket — essential gear for a journey down a murky and sometimes turbulent river. This book is, at the least, a means to test the waters from the safety of your easy chair, or a bible to clutch if you decide to take the plunge.

Acknowledgments

The authors would like to thank the many people who have contributed their time and expertise to this book. First, our deepest gratitude goes to the hospital executives and physicians who have struggled to make their practice acquisitions succeed and have "made it through the rain." From those whom we have helped, we have also learned a great deal. Without them, this book would not have been possible.

Our sincere thanks also go to Susan W. Wallner, a consultant at Amicus, Inc., for coauthoring chapter 6 on practice evaluation; to Katherine Glafkides, an associate at Epstein Becker Stromberg & Green, for her valued contributions to chapter 8 on agreements; and to Rex S. Levering, executive vice-president of Oklahoma Healthcare Corporation, for coauthoring chapters 1 and 9.

In addition, we wish to express our appreciation to Fran Simon Wayne, a consultant at Amicus, Inc., for her assistance in editing selected chapters and in writing the preface. Special thanks are due to Dana Helms, June Kraemer, and Norma Hashinger at Amicus, Inc., for their tireless efforts in typing, retyping, and polishing many chapters of the manuscript.

Finally, a debt of gratitude is owed to Norma Singer Portnoy for her understanding and support through her husband's metamorphosis to author and editor.

Chapter 1

The Strategy of Practice Acquisition

Philip A. Newbold and Rex S. Levering

Where does practice acquisition fit in your organization's plan for physician marketing and practice enhancement programs? Is your hospital already committed to an acquisition strategy, or do you view this wildfire phenomenon as a short-term fad? Hospital executives across the United States are suddenly confronted with overnight changes in practice ownership, radical shifts in physician loyalty, and threatened losses of millions of dollars in annual revenues. The most important question is whether your organization is in the role of activist/aggressor or, instead, observes practice acquisitions by your toughest competitor.

Although many policymakers will elect not to fire the first shot, few hospital executives will escape the practice acquisition game in the next decade. You too will move from the sidelines onto the playing field when a major medical group or an active admitting physician affiliated with your staff entertains a firm offer from a competing hospital.

Considering a Practice Acquisition Strategy

In tackling the practice acquisition question, executives wrestle with issues that are pragmatic, philosophical, and even ethical. Will most physician practices be owned or managed by hospitals (or their affiliate corporations) by 1995? Will productivity and quality be sacrificed as physicians give up their independence and fee-for-service incomes to gain economic security and unload practice management headaches?

For a growing number of entrepreneurial physicians and multispecialty clinics, a practice acquisition strategy should also be considered instead of the usual practice of recruiting a new partner. Physicians have found that forming group practices or networks of practices can have several advantages over solo practice and can offer a hedge against an increasingly uncertain future. Practice acquisitions are intended for any organization or individual who sees a more secure and productive future in growing with already established practices and office settings.

After starting a practice acquisition program, you need to consider some additional questions. For example, how can any organization so dependent on physicians control the pace and scope of the program? Can any executive turn away from offers to sell by "loyal" physicians who have learned their market value as a direct result of the early acquisitions made by their own institution?

Furthermore, how can your hospital carve out policies that treat staff physicians who wish to sell both fairly and evenly while protecting scarce capital dollars? In today's fiercely competitive market, executives are widely divided on the issue. For every CEO who touts the benefits of his or her practice acquisition program, the authors know an equally experienced counterpart who can recount the problems and pitfalls of practice acquisitions. This same difference of opinion can be found in communities across the country as well as in the whole movement in economic joint ventures between hospitals and physicians. In short, the strategies must fit your local community, hospital, and medical staff. There is no one recipe for success.

When you first consider whether a practice acquisition program is right for your health care organization, you should take some time to define for your medical staff and governing body exactly what an acquisition means. In some instances, it may only mean the acquisition of hard assets, such as the office building and improvements, the equipment, and the furnishings. In other instances, an acquisition may mean that the office staff becomes employees of the hospital as well as the physician. There is a wide range of options in practice acquisition programs (see chapter 4), and each health care organization should tailor individual practice opportunities according to a complex and interrelated set of acquisition strategies.

Benefits for the Hospital

Practice acquisitions are aggressive and high-risk ventures at best. At worst, they can topple the careers of top-level executives and set off costly and disruptive counteractions by the acquiring hospital's wounded competitor. Considering the risk, why tackle this strategy at all?

For the winning organization, a successful acquisition program can be the bold stroke that gains the decisive competitive edge, increases market share, and secures financial stability. A few enthusiasts suggest practice acquisition as the logical solution to their hospital's survival and the entire control issue over loosely organized physician practices. These people feel that the informal, loose referral patterns can be controlled or influenced more by actually owning the primary care providers than by relying on more indirect and tenuous lines of referrals.

The principal motivations of hospitals or health care organizations that have pioneered this strategy are:

- *Retaining physicians already on staff.* Many acquisitions are triggered by the threatened loss of a major medical practice or group already active on the hospital staff. The objective is simply to hold on to the loyalties and patient referrals of the physicians who intend to sell. Lacking a market value offer by the hospital, this practice or group is a prime candidate for selling to a competing hospital or medical group.
- *Expanding market share.* For the hospital economist, the acquisition makes business sense. It promises added market share and added income if the buying hospital also earns the loyalty and patient admissions and referrals of the acquired physician or medical group.
- *Aiding the practice in transition.* For the hospital willing to assist its most senior physicians, buying the practice in transition preserves its patient base and makes the hospital an active partner in recruiting a new practitioner.
- *Assisting a practice to expand.* Hospital capital can provide the muscle that an established medical group may be unwilling or unable to invest to provide a more comprehensive and competitive range of programs, services, and facilities.

Benefits for the Physician

When practice acquisition programs succeed, how do the selling physicians benefit? For physicians who embrace the idea, a top-ranking (although always understated) goal is to "cash in" on the asset values they have created through years of practice development. Whether they label the opportunity as "goodwill," "blue sky," or "future business considerations," physicians eager to sell nearly always see *an opportunity to liquidate an asset,* that is, their own practice. When major journals read by most physicians feature cover story headlines and cite huge amounts paid for goodwill (usually by your local hospital), you can be certain that large dollar signs flash in the minds of most of your medical staff members. Building the practice has been the life's work of these physicians, and their emotional investment is quite heavy— so are their expectations and definitions of practice value.

Ensured levels of professional income and economic security are also high on the list of physician goals and may or may not fit into the plans of the buying hospital. Many hospitals have learned that physician productivity and practice revenues frequently drop when physician incomes are guaranteed and the appropriate financial incentives are not in place.

Finally, many physicians are more determined than ever to *pass their practice management headaches on to others*. These physicians yearn to return to the basics of medical practice and patient care. Federal and state bureaucracies, as well as king-sized paper jungles introduced by health maintenance organizations (HMOs), preferred provider organizations (PPOs), and large insurers, have driven thousands of physicians to either shift those burdens to others or retire early. Furthermore, the costs of medical malpractice insurance and the new competitive threats from large corporations contribute to a more complicated and more uncertain future for the practicing physician.

In summary, the one sound economic foundation for long-term practice ownership and management by hospitals and health care systems is to strengthen the practice—to strengthen physician productivity and loyalty and increase practice income and patient volume—and to ensure a steady flow of patients to the hospital or its admitting physicians. Chapter 2 discusses the consideration of practice acquisition in more detail.

Planning for a Successful Acquisition

All practice acquisitions should be undertaken in concert with a well-defined and broadly integrated strategic business plan for the hospital or health care organization. It is the strategic plan that drives the practice enhancement and acquisition process. The strategic plan provides the broad guidance for choosing which practices are most strategic to the hospital and which set of acquisition strategies is likely to be most successful and rewarding. A hospital without a good strategic plan is like a large ship without a rudder in a changing current. Time invested at the front end of the planning process always pays rich dividends during periods of rapid change and chaos later on. Chapter 3 elaborates on the function and elements of an acquisition plan grounded in a hospital's strategic business plan.

As part of the planning process, hospitals need to consider a number of questions:

- Can senior management make good on a platform that promises to strengthen the practice? What enhancement tools, management skills, and marketing resources are available for this purpose within the hospital system?
- How will the transaction affect the physician's hospital admitting practices? Does the physician retain his or her independent professional judgment in seeking the best care for patients, or will the expectations of the buying hospital lead to conflicts between buyer and seller?
- How will the acquisition affect the rest of the physicians on the medical staff, especially those who refer patients to the practice? Will the

staff support the senior management in the po
ing the first acquisition?

- How will the senior management respond to the
  physicians who now expect the corporation
  practices?

These questions are consistently controversial and almost always present legal,
political, and ethical issues. Moreover, practice acquisition focuses on only
one dimension of a balanced physician marketing and practice enhancement program. Effective management intent on excellence in physician marketing and practice enhancement should consider a total spectrum of
strategies for physician recruitment, retention, and practice building. Chapter
8 discusses the details of various sorts of strategies designed to enhance the
physician practice.

A Four-Phased Physician Marketing and Practice Enhancement Program

One model, successfully developed and applied by a leading regional health
care system in the central states, offers a four-phased program for physician marketing and practice enhancement:

1. Basic marketing and enhancement services
2. Physician recruitment strategies
3. Joint ventures and contract management services
4. Acquisition of physician practices

These four phases present a range of strategies along a continuum of broadly
defined physician marketing and practice enhancement activities. Hospitals
may move gradually from some of the more conservative strategies to those
that are more aggressive, or a few hospitals may adopt some of the more
aggressive strategies right away because of pressing competitive market
conditions.

Each phase of the model carries its own level of risks and rewards. Figure
1.1 shows that practice acquisition is the most aggressive strategy but offers
the greatest potential for reward. It also requires heavier cash investment
and commits the hospital to carry the overhead cost of practice management and marketing resources. Executives seeking a more conservative
approach can initiate a wide variety of marketing and enhancement services that consume fewer capital dollars, incur less risk, and perhaps achieve
the same economic benefit if well done.

Figure 1.1. Physician Marketing and Practice Enhancement Strategies

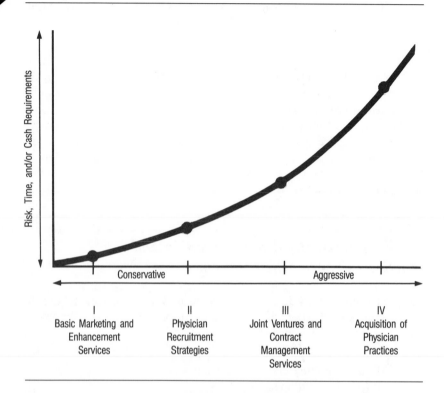

Basic Marketing and Enhancement Services

Before resources are allocated for practice acquisition, managers should carefully assess the practice's fit with the organization's culture as well as the organization's state of readiness with complementary programs for marketing, physician recruitment, and joint ventures. You can quickly assess your state of readiness by undertaking a brief self-examination aided by the checklist of services in figure 1.2. Before embarking on practice acquisitions, you should consider having half or more of the services in the figure operating successfully.

Each service in figure 1.2 strengthens the hospital's preparation for undertaking a practice acquisition strategy, and many services are prerequisites for demonstrating to physicians how acquired practices can benefit from affiliation with the hospital. Capabilities for physician referral programs, public relations and advertising, and market analysis all help to attract physicians interested in selling to a hospital or system. Such services can be used

Figure 1.2.   Checklist for Basic Marketing and Enhancement Services

Among the services listed here that are not in place in your hospital, which ones are essential to make your practice acquisition program successful?

	In Place	Planned
Physician referral program	☐	☐
Public relations and advertising for physicians	☐	☐
Speakers bureau	☐	☐
Orientation programs for new physicians and their office staffs	☐	☐
Seminars and education programs for practice enhancement	☐	☐
Office staff training	☐	☐
Marketing studies and assistance	☐	☐
Group purchasing arrangements	☐	☐
Consulting services	☐	☐
Newcomer services	☐	☐
Physician liaison representative	☐	☐

by senior management to build its early credibility and communicate its expertise to potential acquisition prospects. Without an organized plan to build and expand the practice, executives should think twice before proceeding with the acquisition.

Physician Recruitment Strategies

Organized physician recruitment is the second phase in your hospital's program for physician marketing and practice enhancement. Whether you are operating a 75-bed facility in a rural community or a major metropolitan medical center, you can ensure that your hospital will thrive tomorrow if you have a carefully thought-out physician recruitment program in place today.

Even in the present competitive environment, with physician surpluses in many specialties and in many communities, physician recruitment programs are the lifeblood of any hospital's future; for rapidly declining utilization levels mean more and more physicians will be needed to support the hospital's existing inpatient base. Whether physician recruitment is a highly structured, well-broadcast program supplemented with strong financial incentives or a quietly conducted, informal campaign to strengthen weak links in the medical staff, winning hospitals are more active than ever in physician recruitment programs.

In a real sense, physician recruitment and retention determines the hospital's product distribution system of the future. A hospital that operates without a physician recruitment plan would be like the Chrysler Corporation's managing without an organized system for building and maintaining a strong dealer network. Physician recruitment is so central to every hospital's future success, that it warrants both a carefully developed plan and the involvement of managers at the very top of the organization.

In essence, senior management should follow four steps when planning physician recruitment programs:

1. *Obtain medical staff acceptance and board support for a recruitment plan.* Among voluntary hospitals, the organized medical staff frequently participates in formulating recruitment strategy and policy. A strong, vocal staff may set upper and lower limits on senior management's recruitment ambitions. Although recruitment policy among for-profit hospital systems is governed by slightly different criteria, most executives agree that medical staff leadership and support are the foundation of a successful physician recruitment program. Failing to involve physician leadership in advance inevitably undermines medical staff acceptance and jeopardizes all senior management's past efforts to build medical staff trust and loyalty. Board support is also necessary to ensure that proper legal and tax issues are considered, especially as changes occur in the tax codes and as regulatory pressures increase. The board-approval process should allow for quick and expeditious decisions so that senior management can make commitments and present a competitive financial offer in a timely fashion.

2. *Design a plan that is compatible with medical staff attitudes and the culture of the organization.* The plan should determine which types of physician practices are needed, how many, the time schedule for the acquisition, and resource requirements. In shaping your recruitment plan, you have a wide variety of excellent choices. Experience gained by executives in the late 1970s and early 1980s provides time-tested ideas and a wealth of recruitment tools ranging from hospital-sponsored practice development and consultation services to total practice financing and management. Figure 1.3 lists programs that offer proven results in many major medical centers. Be sure to include transitional strategies that assist a senior practitioner to bring in a new, younger partner so that the hospital does not lose the practice when the physician finally retires.

3. *Obtain review and concurrence by top-notch legal counsel.* In the tax-exempt sector, programs must be structured to avoid the risk of inurement under current Internal Revenue Service policy and the risk of fraud and abuse violations under Medicare rules and regulations. These risks are discussed in chapter 5.

Figure 1.3. Checklist for Physician Recruitment Programs

	In Place	Planned
Practice development business planning	☐	☐
Financial needs assessment	☐	☐
Assistance with purchasing or leasing office equipment	☐	☐
Loan guarantees	☐	☐
Part-time employment	☐	☐
Compensation advances under hospital-managed practices	☐	☐
Medical office building strategies	☐	☐
Education and research assistance	☐	☐
Access to professional liability insurance	☐	☐
Relocation assistance	☐	☐
Practice transition for senior physicians	☐	☐

4. *Present the plan to the board for adoption and funding.* If possible, obtain discretionary spending authority within defined limits so that senior management can proceed effectively and in a timely fashion. It should not be necessary to bring every single recruitment package through a long and complicated approval process. A small committee of the board can be used to monitor these financial arrangements and assure the board and medical staff that the hospital's resources are being used in an effective and appropriate manner.

Many leading hospital executives who steer away from practice acquisition strategies are, instead, aggressive in their physician recruitment programs. For example, one executive of a rural, for-profit hospital attributed his hospital's recent turnaround to successful physician recruitment programs. This executive is convinced his hospital invests less capital and achieves higher returns through recruitment of new physicians than through buying established practices.

Another example of an aggressive physician recruiter is a major regional medical center in the central United States that successfully affiliated with 15 physicians during the first year of its private practice development program. This institution has enjoyed strong medical staff support from the earliest stages of planning because of the medical staff's involvement in shaping the program. Senior management also made it clear from the outset that this medical center desires to give priority to established physicians who wish to expand their practices. A lesson from this example is that staff opinion leaders are less likely to object to the hospital's program when senior management demonstrates that it will extend recruitment assistance to established staff members who wish to add new associates.

Joint Ventures and Contract Management Services

The third phase of a comprehensive program for physician marketing and practice enhancement—that is, joint ventures and contract management relationships with physicians—is for many hospital management teams a major strategy for attracting and retaining medical staff loyalty and for closing the patient referral loop. Proven success in joint ventures and contract management is also an excellent platform from which to launch a practice acquisition program. A multitude of new joint venture and contract management relationships have evolved, especially among hospital systems committed to ambulatory care and after-care services. Such services include:

- Computed tomography and magnetic resonance imaging
- Clinical laboratory
- Outpatient surgery
- Durable medical equipment
- Home intravenous therapy; total parenteral nutrition
- Mobile lithotripsy
- Mobile mammography
- Chronic dialysis
- Skilled nursing facility
- Urgent care facility
- Medical office buildings
- Managed care programs (HMOs and PPOs)
- Sports medicine programs
- Outpatient mental health clinics

Joint Ventures

Ernst and Whinney's survey of 400 hospitals, "Health Care Joint Ventures Survey Results" (1985), revealed that from the hospital's perspective nearly 75 percent of hospital joint ventures were precipitated by the desire to increase market share whereas only 25 percent were formed principally to develop new sources of capital. Alternate delivery systems (PPOs and HMOs), medical office buildings, freestanding surgery centers, and imaging centers are examples of joint ventures that are shared with physicians to strengthen market share. Hospital joint ventures involving nonphysician partners are more likely to be formed to develop new sources of capital.

The most popular ventures by far among physicians are those tied directly to the physician's office practice. Driven by wanting to strengthen their practice incomes, private practice physicians most frequently invest their own cash in alternate delivery systems (principally PPOs and HMOs) and medical office building partnerships. Hospitals have also found these ventures to be the most effective method to support high levels of bed occupancy. In contrast, ventures limited to return-on-investment objectives that do not contribute patients to physician office practices (such as nursing homes, imaging centers, and durable medical equipment ventures) may attract only nominal numbers of physician investors.

Institutions most experienced in joint ventures consider the major advantage of such ventures to be building a climate of trust and demonstrated willingness to share the financial rewards with physicians. One executive who has presided over nearly 20 joint ventures now believes the loyalty gained by making venture opportunities available to key physicians is the greatest single benefit of joint venture offerings. When physicians understand the hospital's good-faith intent, the perception itself pays long-term dividends in medical staff support whether or not these physicians invest in the project.

Contract Management Services

In yet another form of joint venture, many hospitals have entered the contract management business. Some hospitals are reversing the usual format by placing qualified physician entrepreneurs in the role of contract managers. Today's large hospital typically has an entire division devoted to managing physician practices, urgent care centers, or hospital-owned primary care center satellites. These entities operate as contract management organizations. Expert practice managers, undiluted by assignments in hospital operations, are essential to make practice acquisitions work, and practicing physicians with good administrative skills can bring a crucial new dimension to this competitive arena.

Executives who were trained to think that physicians cannot manage are today frequently finding themselves executing contracts with physicians as "managers." By establishing occupational medicine programs, freestanding surgery centers, and sports medicine, more executives are learning that the right physicians may be the best qualified and most entrepreneurial managers for these small business enterprises. Ventures suited for physician management, for example, sports medicine and occupational medicine programs, may also present an opportunity to strengthen the institution's patient referral network.

When developing contract management services, today's executive is confronted with a host of alternatives for incorporating computer linkages between physician offices and the hospital. Opinions remain widely divided on this issue as many aggressive medical centers move to install personal computers in the offices of 50, 100, or more physicians. Whatever your organization's policy on computer networks is, you should ask four key questions when choosing a course of action:

- What market research has been conducted to determine the services your medical staff would value most?
- Does your hospital information system offer the capacity to link with computers in medical staff offices without a major capital investment?
- If your organization is 501(C)(3) tax exempt, has legal counsel determined there are no issues of inurement created by your proposed program?
- Have you determined that changing technology will not quickly obsolete the office computer hardware, software, and hospital office link contemplated for your network?

Acquisition of Physician Practices

Many organizations believe that experience in the first three phases of physician marketing and practice enhancement — basic marketing and enhancement services, physician recruitment, and joint ventures and contract management services — is a requisite for success in the fourth and most aggressive phase, practice acquisition. But other organizations may consider buying practices without first having a comprehensive marketing and enhancement program in place. Such organizations may be responding to unexpected opportunities (or necessity) that allow no time to implement a carefully thought-out program in advance. Although these organizations may succeed with practice acquisition, they would be wise to carefully assess their ability to enhance the practice before rather than after the deal is closed. One question they should ask themselves is whether they have any marketing and management services they can offer to the practice.

Organizations without a comprehensive marketing and enhancement program should also assess their ability to meet physician expectations. Many selling physicians cling to the notion that hospitals have the marketing muscle and management talent to increase patient visits, reduce accounts receivable, and assume the headaches of practice management regardless of the facts. When asked why practice acquisitions fail, one executive pinpointed the gap between physician expectations and actual results as the most frequent cause of major breakdown after the closing. Executives should be certain that the expectations of selling physicians are realistic.

Before acquiring a physician's practice, the management team should seek answers to the following questions:

- What resources are already available within the hospital to support a practice acquisition strategy?
- Are hospital management and marketing skills transferable to medical practice management?
- What additional human resources are required, and at what cost?

- Can the hospital increase physician practice revenues sufficiently to both amortize the capital investment and cover the added overhead of the practice management team?
- What financial policy will guide practice acquisition and management? Can the hospital amortize its cash investment with net cash flows from the practice? If not, how will investment capital be recovered?
- What criteria will guide senior management in selecting acquisition candidates?
- In developing the economic model, what are the targeted financial returns as measured by practice cash flows and additional inpatient admissions?
- What valuation methods will be adopted for goodwill, accounts receivable, and office equipment?
- Will medical office real estate be purchased as part of the acquisition program or leased from the current owner?
- What political problems will practice acquisitions generate? How will senior management respond?
- What scenario does senior management project for the long-term future of practice acquisitions? Will the acquisitions program be limited to a very few practices, or will the acquisition option be available to the entire medical staff?
- What organizational model will be effective for establishing the practice acquisition and management team within the health care system or hospital?
- What legal issues does practice acquisition present? Has legal counsel endorsed the program?

Seeking answers to these questions in advance of your first acquisition will help secure the success of the program. Chapters 6 and 7 demonstrate how successful organizations have handled these questions.

The senior management should also carefully think through sensitive ethical issues in advance of making any offers to purchase:

- Are the goals of the intended partnership built on mutually understood and compatible expectations? Does the hospital understand the physician's obligation to refer patients to the best-qualified physicians and hospitals? Will physicians in the acquired practice transfer their loyalties from one hospital to another and from former colleagues to new referral physicians? If the hospital affiliation will be a new experience for these physicians, have professional relationships with attending staff been tested in advance? How will the hospital demonstrate its ability to make the physician's practice grow? In short, have the parties to the transaction assured themselves that all professional

and philosophical issues are in balance with the terms of the purchase transaction?

- What are the quality of care impacts of these new business ownership combinations? Will the physician's advocacy for his or her patient
be altered by the new economic arrangements? Will the hospital's
management of the practice or its employment practices increase or
detract from high-quality patient care? What quality-of-care measurement devices should be in place to assure the hospital's governing body that quality of care has improved as a result of the hospital's
ownership? How can the collective resources of the hospital be lever-
aged to improve the quality of care in remote office practices?
- What are the expectations of the parties regarding the flow of patient
admissions? Does the physician retain free choice of physicians and
hospitals under the terms of the sale agreement? At stake here are
not only the ethics of the relationship but also Medicare fraud and
abuse regulations, professional liability, and possible violations of state
statutes. In addition, will conflicts of interest be a problem with the
medical staff? What is the best way to inform patients as to these
new ownership issues and potential economic impacts? One family
medicine physician on the brink of acquisition by a major medical
center avoided a conflict by alerting the buyer that his cardiac patient
referrals would continue to go to the stronger cardiology program
at a competing medical center.

Programs built on the premise of capturing all patient admissions from
the acquired practice may be unrealistic and may jeopardize the hospital's
standing under both federal and state law. You should keep in mind that
the vast majority of practice acquisitions involve primary care physicians
since specialists' practices rely on established referral patterns that can be
severely damaged or altered if involved with medical staff opposition to
acquisition strategies.

Before beginning a practice acquisition negotiation, you should test your
readiness. The checklist in figure 1.4 can be used to aid your self-evaluation.

Pros and Cons of Practice Acquisition for the Hospital

To summarize this introduction to practice acquisition, we have included
a list of some advantages and disadvantages (see figure 1.5). Because practice acquisition is a high-stakes strategy and is often controversial, we have
listed each major benefit and its risk to the hospital.

Gaining and protecting market share ranks high in every practice acquisition strategy. Practice acquisition programs that promise to survive and
thrive beyond the short-term trend are those that are structured to:

Figure 1.4. Checklist for Practice Acquisition Programs

	In Place or Completed	Planned
Practice management expertise	☐	☐
Determination of staffing needs	☐	☐
Program objectives and expected results	☐	☐
Financial policy and capital investment allocations	☐	☐
Criteria adopted for practice acquisition	☐	☐
Valuation methods	☐	☐
Medical staff considerations	☐	☐
Short-term and long-term strategy	☐	☐
Organizational model	☐	☐
Consideration of legal and ethical issues	☐	☐

Figure 1.5. Pros and Cons of Practice Acquisition for the Hospital

For Acquisition	Against Acquisition
Gains market share	Risks loss of medical staff support
Takes physicians away from competitors	May trigger an acquisition program by a tough competitor
Builds a system of hospital-owned practices	Requires major capital outlays
Recruits new physicians to the institution	May trigger demands to purchase from less desirable acquisition candidates who are already established members of the staff
Controls physician admitting patterns	May violate legal and ethical mandates and state and federal laws
Enhances physician practices	Requires committed marketing, management, and financial resources

- Increase patient practice volume, expand the physician base, and increase net cash flows
- Amortize capital investment through increased practice revenues
- Strengthen the overall medical staff organization

Remember that a physician acquisition strategy is a patient acquisition strategy, so where practice referrals are directed is a key issue in the entire planning and preparation process.

Organizations embracing the practice acquisition strategy should carefully set out (1) their criteria for selecting acquisition candidates and (2) the impact of these criteria on both capital outlays and medical staff relationships. For example, does it make more sense for your institution to acquire the practices of your most loyal physicians first or, instead, the non-admitters who currently favor a competitor? Or is your hospital's position better served by a strategy that focuses initially on physicians that split their admissions between two or more hospitals? In almost every case, consultation with medical staff leaders in advance of searching for acquisition candidates is in your organization's best interest.

If a hospital adopts the four-phased model set forth in this chapter, it has the opportunity to develop a comprehensive marketing and enhancement program in which practice acquisition is only the final step. One advantage of this model is that when a practice acquisition program is undertaken, the hospital has already gained experience in basic marketing and enhancement services, physician recruitment, and joint ventures and contract management services. This experience can be readily applied to making the acquired practice successful, and the hospital is in the best position for reaping the greatest rewards of a practice acquisition program.

Chapter 2

Why Hospitals Buy Practices, and Why Physicians Sell Them

Steven Portnoy

The health care delivery system is rapidly changing. This change has become so dramatic over the past five or six years as to cause some private practices and hospitals to merge their assets and destinies. While, in certain cases, large group practices have purchased hospitals, in most cases hospitals are purchasing solo and group practices.

With the organization, delivery, and financing of health care services evolving so significantly across the country, hospitals and physicians in private practice are exploring new techniques for ensuring survival and growth. Hospitals are becoming multifaceted health care systems participating in all levels and locales of care. In vying for their "piece of the market," an increasing number of hospitals are acquiring private physicians' practices. Such an acquisition strategy enables hospitals to move further into the local health care delivery scene and gives the selling physicians the resources for ensuring the viability of their practices.

Hospital Motivations to Acquire Practices

Unlike situations in the past where hospitals have helped young physicians to finance the purchase of retiring physicians' practices, hospital acquisition programs today reflect a flurry of new activity, particularly with primary care practitioners, whereby hospitals are buying those practices and practice sites and are often hiring the physicians as full-time employees of, or contractors to, the hospital. The willingness of successful private practitioners to consider this kind of arrangement, and to change their status from independent entrepreneurs to hospital employees or contractors, may represent a significant alteration in the relationship between hospitals and physicians. Although the impact of this new level of interface remains to be seen, the benefits to the hospital are many.

Controlling Admissions and Referrals

As hospitals position themselves to survive, they are more aggressively competing for patients, for physicians, and for resources. Institutions that have become involved in the purchase of doctors' practices are finding acquisition to be a very potent competitive tool. Recognizing that the vast majority of patients come to the hospital through their physicians' practices, hospitals are seeking to protect those sources of admissions and referrals and to expand them. Acquisition enables them to control access to the health care delivery system and ensure a steady flow of patients to the hospital.

Traditionally, without owning and operating a particular doctor's office practice, a hospital could not expect to receive some (or all) of the patients from that doctor. It has always been a matter of choice for the doctor (not usually the patient and never the hospital) as to where the patient would be sent.

As an employee (or a contractor) of a hospital, the physician practicing in an "owned practice" will most likely send the patient to the hospital that owns the practice, assuming that the necessary services are available and that they are of adequate quality to meet the needs of each patient being hospitalized. Hospitals should be very careful not to require doctors to admit patients needing hospitalization to their facility if they are unable to provide adequate, high-quality care in the area of need. The legal issues relating to requiring admissions or referrals from doctors will be dealt with in chapter 5 of this book.

Even where a practice is owned by a hospital, the patients still have the opportunity to determine where they will be admitted. However, in order to go to a different hospital, the patient may have to find a different doctor if the hospital's acquisition program does not allow for multiple staff appointments.

Protecting and Expanding Market Share

Obviously, then, one of the major motivations for hospitals to acquire physicians' practices relates to market share and the consequent protection of, and increase in, hospital revenues. Depending on the extent to which a hospital chooses to participate in acquisition, a hospital can protect its current markets to maintain the status quo, increase market share in communities already being served, or expand into new geographic areas. If the acquiring hospital is already the hospital of choice for a physician whose practice is being acquired, there will be limited potential for expanding market share or developing new geographic areas. Acquiring such practices would, however, serve to ensure that patients currently coming from the practice will continue to do so and that the physician will not shift his or her activities to another hospital.

Hospitals that participate in practice acquisition activities purely as a defensive strategy often believe that they should do it before it is done to them by the hospital down the street. It is not unusual to find a hospital buying doctors' practices after hearing rumors that a competitor hospital is about to do so, or after losing one of the hospital's active, loyal practitioners through a sale to the competitor. Unfortunately, it is also not unusual for a hospital to be unaware that one of its important practices has been acquired.

In cases where the acquired practice has traditionally split its admissions and referrals between two or more hospitals, the acquisition enables the hospital to increase its share from that physician's practice and, therefore, from that community's market. If the practice being purchased has never before admitted or referred patients to the acquiring hospital, the hospital can obtain an overnight increase in market share through the conversion of an active private practice into a thriving hospital satellite. Acquiring high-quality, busy practices can provide the quickest return on investment of almost any competitive strategy available to hospitals. The result is an immediate shift in market share from one hospital to another.

Influencing HMOs and PPOs

One reason that is being increasingly recognized as a benefit of acquisition strategies is the control hospitals gain over the gatekeepers sought out by health maintenance organizations (HMOs) and preferred provider organizations (PPOs). Ownership of a geographically well-positioned set of primary care offices can enable a hospital to have much influence over negotiations with managed care organizations. This would be at least of equal benefit to hospitals wishing to develop their own HMOs or PPOs.

As a result of acquisition, a hospital also has a greater ability to influence the practice activities of primary care gatekeepers who work for the hospital. This influence helps solve a major problem for hospitals affiliated with HMOs, which has been an inability to contain unnecessary tests, referrals, and so forth with gatekeepers who have become hospital employees or contractors. The hospital contracting with an HMO or PPO is better able to effect change in the way those gatekeepers practice and refer to specialists. This control, in turn, affects the price of the hospital's services. The acquiring hospital, however, must know how to influence practice style without negatively affecting the ability of the physician to provide needed services for the patient. The incentive is increased efficiency and productivity in caring for patients both within the practice and in the hospital.

Attracting More Profitable Business

Hospitals should not overlook, as a motivation to become involved in acquisition, the increased ability to improve payer mix or diagnosis-related group (DRG) mix. Simply put, an acquisition program can attract more favorable practices from a DRG or payer mix standpoint. Hospitals seeking to find more efficient practitioners or to attract more business from physicians providing clinical services that are money-makers at the hospital rather than money-losers can reap many rewards through the acquisition of appropriate practices.

Although practice ownership can enable hospitals to monitor and influence practice overhead and the use of hospital services, one note of caution should be kept in mind: It is not at all unusual for a hospital to increase a practice's costs as a result of acquisition. This results from the hospital's inexperience with managing private practices, and doing so efficiently, and from the hospital's desire to "strengthen" the practice and therefore introduce new and expensive equipment, operational systems, or expanded staffing into the practice.

Developing Group Practices

The development of group practices is another motivation for hospitals considering the acquisition strategy. Across the country there is growing interest in forming affiliations between practices. This trend is occurring for a variety of reasons, not the least of which is for the sharing of overhead and for mutual self-defense to ensure survival.

Increasingly, physicians are open to involving hospitals as sources of technical support in advising them on how to form groups. Such support ranges from assistance with evaluating the feasibility of a merger or other form of affiliation with another practice to assistance in implementing the affiliation. Ventures between such practices may result in the need for a new office building or for services to be provided for the new group, such as computer systems or laboratory X-ray services. Many hospitals are interested in participating in such opportunities.

Hospitals being invited by their physicians to assist them in group practice development and hospitals wishing to encourage their doctors to develop groups should give serious consideration to practice acquisition as a tool for building group practices. If a hospital believes that a key to the future survival of its active and loyal doctors' practices is the development of groups, certainly the merger of some of the practices can be facilitated through acquisition.

Once the hospital owns the individual practices, it can more easily influence the involved physicians to participate together in a group. This is particularly true when new physicians, who are more open to group practice, are brought in to take over from the selling physicians, who are retiring. However, it is often the case that the selling physicians intend to remain with the new, expanded practice. In this case, they usually enter into the acquisition contract with the understanding that they will be expected to practice closely with other hospital physicians whose practices have also been acquired.

Accomplishing Product Line and Manpower Objectives

A hospital may also wish to acquire physicians' practices when it sees practice acquisition as a tool for achieving the objectives of its product line strategies or its medical staff development plan. Where a hospital has identified product lines to be strengthened or newly developed (requiring the addition of more or different specialists), or where it has identified gaps in the current medical staff (requiring the recruitment of additional doctors), a practice acquisition program can be very beneficial.

While the majority of acquired practices seem to be in the area of primary care, some hospitals are purchasing specialty practices previously not available or active on the staff. Certainly, a hospital's ability to attract specialists (even if not acquired) is enhanced if it maintains an active acquisition program for primary care practices and can influence those doctors to refer to specialists who have newly arrived on staff. Any chief executive who has attempted to recruit new specialists to his or her staff knows that such doctors are reluctant to accept the offer if they are concerned that they will be unable to break into long-established primary care referral networks. If a hospital has an acquisition program for primary care practices, this program creates a greater opportunity for referral patterns to develop to newly attracted specialists. All of this assumes that the quality-of-care expectations of both the primary care and specialty physicians will be satisfactory to both groups.

Expanding Ambulatory Care Services and Developing New Ventures

Hospitals seeking new markets for ambulatory care services realize several benefits from participating in practice acquisition. It is much easier to expand the hospital's market for physical therapy, laboratory, durable medical equipment (DME), home care, and other services if the hospital controls the distribution system. While currently not seen by the author as an initial motivation for most hospitals to participate in practice acquisition, hospitals that have actively acquired doctors' practices are reaping the rewards of having a broader distribution system under their influence. They no longer have to work as hard to persuade the physicians to refer to their home care agency, to use their DME equipment, to send their patients to (or provide a site for) the hospital's physical therapy or sports medicine programs, and so forth. The physicians are now much more closely linked with that hospital and all of its services.

Practice acquisition also can enable a hospital to undertake new ventures more easily and build the success of those initiatives more rapidly. For example, employed or contracted physicians providing services at hospital-owned primary care offices are much more likely to allow the hospital to develop an industrial medicine program without feeling threatened by that as a competitive activity of the hospital. Whether the industrial medicine venture is a freestanding program unrelated to the acquired doctors' practices, or whether the employed physicians staffing those practices participate in the industrial medicine program, physicians practicing as employees or on contract are more likely to support the success of such a venture.

Physician Motivations to Sell Practices

Although hospitals think in terms of "practice acquisition," physicians think in terms of "practice sale." Hospitals should understand the reasons why more and more doctors are giving serious consideration to selling their practices, for understanding these reasons before approaching a physician can often make the difference between arousing serious interest and alienating the physician.

Doctors are far more willing to seriously explore the sale of their practice to a hospital today than they were even two or three years ago. What was a firm no two years ago is often a reluctantly spoken, or perhaps enthusiastic, yes today. Changing times for physicians in private practice have led to changing minds.

Issues that have made the independent practice of medicine less desirable to some doctors and the alternatives more worth exploring include: tremendous growth in the number of physicians in practice throughout much of the United States; excessive overhead from factors such as major increases in malpractice insurance premiums; competition from HMOs and other providers of health care services for what has traditionally been the province of the private-practicing physician; and unacceptable requirements for time to be spent on practice administration.

Open and honest discussions with physicians who are considering, or who have already consummated, the sale of their practice usually reveal motivations that are both objective and subjective. It is common for a doctor to sell because of both reason and emotion. To understand some of these motivations, the discussion is organized according to physician age groupings. Even though some reasons to sell apply to any age group, there appears to be a commonality among all the motivations cited by older doctors, those in their middle years, and young doctors who have recently graduated from residency programs and who have been in practice only a few years.

Older Physicians

Older physicians of preretirement age who choose to sell their practices to hospitals cite a variety of reasons. One is that the sale of the practice is obviously *an opportunity to make money.* A professional medical practice is also a business. As is the case with any other business owner, a physician finds it appealing to take his or her equity out of the business if the opportunity arises. Years of effort and commitment have gone into building the practice. It is not unreasonable for a physician to wish to be further compensated for all of those years, especially when approaching retirement.

The price that physicians can obtain from a hospital's purchasing their practice is often greater than what they would receive from other physicians' buying them out. Hospitals are more willing to recognize the value of goodwill in a physician's practice and to view the practice as a satellite, offering much growth opportunity through market share expansion and new service development.

Selling to a hospital can be made even more attractive if the practice is located in a medical office building or house that is owned by the physician. Hospitals are often willing to purchase the real estate in addition to the practice, which may not be true of physicians considering purchase of the practice.

It is not unusual to hear an older physician say, "I hear that practices may soon be worthless because of all the changes going on in medicine. I think I'll sell while I can." Having spent a lifetime building a successful practice, a growing number of older doctors are increasingly fearful that the window of opportunity for selling that practice may be closing.

Many preretirement physicians are attracted to hospitals because hospitals offer the potential for lucrative *retirement packages* and future financial security. This is certainly true if the physician is willing to spend several years at the practice following the sale. This will allow time to introduce a new, young physician to the patients and thus ensure the smooth transition of the practice to the hospital. Selling physicians and acquiring hospitals are together devising retirement packages that are of reasonable cost to the hospital and that relieve physicians of financial worries in later years. Many of those doctors feel that if they had been unable to sell the practice to a hospital or another physician, their financial status would have been significantly changed upon retirement, and they would not have been able to offer the same financial security to their families.

Some older doctors choose to sell their practices to hospitals for *health reasons.* If health is suffering and the amount of time a physician can devote to patients is decreasing, the physician's income is also decreasing. The future stability and viability of the practice may soon be in question. Selling one's practice to a hospital can result in an additional physician being made available to fill the gaps in hours of office and hospital coverage and, therefore, maintain the long-term viability of the practice. The patients therefore have the impression that the physician has chosen to expand for their benefit and for the long-term growth of the practice rather than that the doctor is moving toward retirement and that the patients had better seek medical care elsewhere.

Anyone familiar with private medical practice today knows that the amount of time, energy, and money devoted to the business side of the practice has increased enormously. Most doctors chose medicine as a career in order to provide medical services for the public, not because they wanted to fill out forms and run a business. It is understandable that many older (and younger) physicians would like to rid themselves of the business headaches of private practice. Selling to a hospital can quickly lead to a situation in which an older physician can continue to practice until retirement, with immediate and substantial *relief from the attendant administrative chores.* Many acquiring hospitals are willing to assume responsibility for the administrative side of the practice, freeing the physician to spend most of his or her time caring for patients.

The emotional appeal of a large institution's coming in to *protect the long life of a valued practice* is often a motivation for physicians who sell their practices to a hospital. Most doctors care deeply for the future welfare of their patients and have tried very hard to build a high-quality practice and an outstanding reputation. They have devoted many years responding to the medical needs of their patients. Such physicians can be relieved to find a strong hospital that is building for its own future by making them an offer that will "guarantee continuation of the practice I have built up over all these years." This factor should not be overlooked when approaching physician candidates and trying to interest them in selling.

Some resistance to practice acquisition may come from older doctors who are uncomfortable with the notion of group practice. In fact, the older a physician is, the more likely he or she is a devout believer that solo practice is the only way to practice medicine and that groups of more than two or three physicians, and physicians employed by HMOs or hospitals, are "traitors to the cause." One may wonder how it is possible to approach some of these older doctors successfully as they have long been adherents of the idea of maintaining independence.

On this point, the reader may be interested to know that many older physicians entering negotiations to sell their practices to hospitals make the observation that "no self-respecting physician in private practice would be in anything larger than a two- or three-person group, but . . . now that I am 62 and successful, and with all the changes going on, I am *ready for something other than the private practice of medicine.*" Thus many such doctors perceive the sale of their practice to a hospital to be something other than having "sold out." They have merely decided to leave private practice and take a position with a hospital wishing to convert their private practice into a satellite facility providing health care services to the community. They have not decided to join a hospital and other new physicians in a corporately held private practice group. This may appear to be a subtle psychological difference, but for some doctors it makes the concept of the impending change more palatable. Hence this difference should be understood by the acquiring hospital.

Hospitals buying practices from older doctors should be especially cautious about finding out whether a "preretiree" is actually a "retiree." It would be disastrous for the practice if the physician suddenly lost interest and reduced his or her work hours and effort following the date of the sale. The change would be felt by the patients, and the practice would quickly lose much of the value that gave rise to the hospital's interest in the first place.

Some older doctors who have been active at a hospital for many years and who have played a role in its growth wish to sell to that institution as one final action they can take to add to the *continued success of the hospital.* These physicians are very loyal and are proud of their affiliation with the hospital. They feel the hospital has done something for them over the years, and they respond favorably to a chance to display their appreciation. Some of these situations result in very inexpensive purchase prices for hospitals.

Doctors in Their Middle Years

Some hospitals make the mistake of believing that no good physician with a booming practice who is 50 years old would have any reason to sell to a hospital. These institutions, if they hear about such a doctor, are skeptical as to whether the practice is really of high quality and is as successful as it appears. They often wonder whether the doctor is hiding something.

It has been this author's experience that there are growing numbers of successful, competent doctors in their middle years who have decided they have very legitimate reasons to sell to a hospital and become employees or contractors. Such doctors often cite the changing health care delivery system as their primary reason. They see the possible sale of their practice as unfortunate but realistic and smart. Although many doctors may wish it were otherwise, they view linkage with a hospital as an intelligent way to *ensure the future viability of their practice* and their future growth within the practice. They view the changes in the health care delivery system as a force to be reckoned with, oftentimes saying, "I see the handwriting on the wall." This is a strategic motivation for selling a practice and is a reflection of their newly evolving vision of the future model of health care delivery.

These doctors do not believe that the independent practitioner maintaining a private practice in the community will have a meaningful role in the future of medical care. They recognize the increased competition with physicians, hospitals, HMOs, and so forth, and they wish to *share the risk* with someone. When they consider their options for so doing, these doctors choose a strong hospital rather than merging with a group practice or working for an HMO. They choose the stability and security that they perceive to come from affiliating with a large organization rather than a small one.

Some doctors in their middle years who choose to sell to a hospital do so for reasons other than defensive ones. It is not unusual to be told by high-quality physicians with very successful private practices (perhaps a small group practice) that they see affiliation with a hospital as a real opportunity to take advantage of the changes in the health care delivery system. They feel they will now be involved with a large organization with far more resources to develop new ventures and expand market share. They are interested in *pooling financial resources* with other acquired physicians and with the hospital to market their practices energetically and to develop multi-specialty and ancillary service centers.

These doctors are not withdrawing from the practice of medicine. They are helping to reconfigure it. Many of them are energetic and enterprising and, in light of the changing world around them, are looking for the best way to continue their past success. They have decided that, for them, that way is by affiliating with a hospital through the sale of their practice.

As is the case with the preretirement physician group, a growing number of doctors in their middle years of practice look forward to *giving up, or reducing, their administrative headaches* through affiliation with a hospital. While some of the same benefits may be achieved by forming a large group practice, these doctors have selected hospital affiliation, often based on the assumption that hospitals have greater resources to help conduct the business side of the practice. Like the older physician, they feel they trained to practice medicine, not administration.

Doctors in their middle years see the opportunity, through a hospital, to achieve economies of scale with other physicians by means of *group purchasing arrangements and other shared services.* They also perceive that a hospital can help them deal more effectively with the increasing financial and legal burdens of medical malpractice.

Some physicians perceive such significant changes coming in the health care delivery system that they feel the only way to *ensure affiliation in the future with a good hospital* will be to have their practice owned by that hospital. They foresee, given the tremendous competition between hospitals and the excessive number of physicians in many metropolitan and suburban communities, that the good hospitals will eventually have totally closed staffs. These physicians view practice acquisition as a guarantee that they are "in" when the staff is closed and when hospitals have the power to choose which physicians they want, rather than physicians choosing their hospitals. These physicians also perceive that the hospitals of the future will devote their resources to ensuring the success of practices in which they have a major investment rather than subsidizing new equipment purchases and joint venture initiatives for physicians on staff whose practices are not satellites of the hospital.

Younger Physicians

Why do young doctors, in practice for only a few years, choose to sell to a hospital? Many such doctors, having been schooled recently in the midst of the current changes in health care delivery, have a very different outlook from their predecessors. While they want to provide medical care to patients and want to make as much money as those who went before them, their expectations of how this can and should be accomplished are different.

Many young doctors who have established practices in the last two or three years, especially in primary care, have become motivated to sell to a hospital as a result of their growing belief that "solo is out." They are finding that a one- or two-person practice, regardless of their qualities or the energies they devote to building the practice, simply *cannot survive in a highly competitive environment.* It has been very difficult for them to hang out the shingle and expand the practice automatically.

The avoidance of solo practice among young doctors is, however, not universally true, for communities needing new primary care doctors still exist. But in many parts of the country, young doctors are finding it very difficult to maintain financial viability in a tremendously competitive marketplace while dealing with increasing overhead. These doctors have encountered the same administrative headaches and growth in overhead as the middle-aged and preretirement physicians but have far fewer resources to deal with them. Thus they are open to affiliating with an organization that can offer *financial resources and administrative support* for their practices.

Generally, younger doctors are more open to the group practice concept. Hospital acquisition of their private practices can often result in merging a solo physician with other doctors (at their site or elsewhere). After having tried practicing by themselves or perhaps with one other physician, many of these young doctors find that they would like to be part of a larger group. This is so for reasons other than financial security, administrative support, and pooling of resources. Younger doctors are discovering that they want to limit their work to Monday through Friday, and they want *reasonable daytime hours,* not nights and weekends. They wish to have greater opportunity to get away from the practice for vacations or educational seminars. They want *less risk* for themselves and their families. They want *shared malpractice protection.* Affiliation with a hospital and with other doctors who have sold their practices to that hospital can offer exactly such an environment.

It appears to this author that the definition of an "acceptable group practice size" for a young doctor seeking to leave solo practice is directly related to the pace of change in the health care delivery system of the community where the doctor is located. In communities that have been a hotbed of competition for a long period of time and that have seen the early evolution of HMOs, PPOs, and other entrepreneurial ventures and alternative delivery systems, physicians are usually more interested in joining a group with a larger number of doctors. Young doctors in Minneapolis, for example, believe they can only be successful in a group practice clinic or as an HMO employee where there are 50 or more physicians involved. In Philadelphia, where change in the health care delivery system has not been as intense for as long as in Minneapolis, many young physicians who believe their chance of success is greater with a group practice define that to mean a three- to five-person group. In other parts of the country, which fall between Philadelphia and Minneapolis in terms of the "age" and pace of change, an acceptable group practice size for young doctors wishing to leave solo practice is between 10 and 30 physicians.

A young physician interested in selling his or her practice to join a group often finds it relatively easy to go one step further and consider hospital ownership as an alternative to group practice. The larger the group in which the physician is willing to participate, the more he or she is an employee rather than an owner/partner. A natural alternative then to joining a group practice would be an affiliation with a stable, high-quality institution through the sale of one's practice to a hospital.

Conclusion

In conclusion, it is clear that hospitals are motivated to buy practices and physicians are motivated to sell them for a great variety of reasons. A careful examination of one's objectives for buying or selling must be undertaken in order to fully understand whether the transaction is likely to result in achieving those objectives.

Chapter 3

Practice Acquisition Planning and Implementation

Steven Portnoy

Practice acquisition is not for everyone. It is, however, a very potent business development strategy for the growing body of hospitals that have prepared themselves to undertake such activities. In most cases, the hospitals pursuing practice acquisition most successfully are those that first tested their readiness to participate. They asked themselves the vital question: "Is my institution, and are my physicians, ready for acquisition?" To assist hospitals considering the development and implementation of an acquisition program, this chapter includes a brief self-test (figure 3.1) to help each hospital evaluate whether it is appropriate for, and currently prepared for, buying doctors' practices.

If you are considering an acquisition program but do not know the answer to some of the questions in figure 3.1 or have answered them no, do not begin to acquire practices. You are not ready! This chapter will help you understand the issues raised in the self-test, and other issues as well, so that you will feel comfortable with acquiring physicians' practices when you are ready to do so.

There are few activities that can be undertaken by a hospital executive and that can lead as quickly to failure and the need to seek new employment as the unplanned acquisition of physicians' practices. However, there are few business development strategies that can result overnight in as substantial an increase in market share for a hospital as can a properly planned and implemented acquisition program.

Acquisition and the Hospital's Strategic Business Plan

A practice acquisition program should be based on a demonstrated need for primary care or specialty practices. Identification of specific objectives

Figure 3.1. Self-Test for Evaluating Hospital Readiness for Practice Acquisition

Is Acquisition for Us and, If So, Are We Ready?

1. With regard to our market area:
   a. Will the people who reside in our community leave their doctor because his or her practice has been purchased by a hospital? [This issue deals with community perceptions and expectations of "their" doctors, "good" doctors, and issues related to health care versus business.]

2. With regard to our hospital and board of trustees:
   a. What percentage of the board is comfortable with the hospital's owning doctors' practices? [This issue deals with the board's view of the mission of the hospital and its organizational culture and ethics. If you do not know the answer to this question, you should find out before embarking on an acquisition program in order to avoid unpleasant surprises later in the game.]
   b. Does our hospital currently have the best structure to support acquired practices legally, operationally, and financially?
   c. With regard to financial requirements, are our board's return-on-investment expectations achievable from new ventures such as acquisitions?
   d. If an acquired practice fails financially, will we have to end our entire acquisition program?

3. With regard to area doctors:
   a. Can we currently list all the practices in our community that are now owned by a hospital, and can we name the hospital that owns each? [If not, you may be incorrectly perceiving that your community does not participate in acquisition, and you may need to know more about what is happening in your medical marketplace.]
   b. Do we know the facts about our medical staff's opinion of practice acquisition? Have we ever surveyed our entire medical staff to obtain that information? Do we know what percentage prefer ownership by a joint venture corporation between the medical staff and hospital?
   c. With regard to medical staff politics on the issue of "who gets what," are we required to have one standard formula to offer to each doctor's practice we want to acquire?
   d. With respect to our medical staff and its relationship to our management team, do our doctors trust management to conduct a practice acquisition program?
   e. Have we invited our medical staff to speak with us about selling before going to another hospital to explore the opportunity? Are any of our active, loyal physicians currently involved in practice-sale discussions with a competitor hospital?

4. With regard to the management team at our hospital:
   a. When it comes to searching for appropriate acquisition candidates and selling those doctors on the concept, do we have the right person available to make the first contact with physicians about selling their practices? What percentage of their time can be devoted exclusively to acquisition activity?
   b. When it comes to evaluating practices that are candidates for acquisition, how many months or years of the candidates' patient and financial records do we want our evaluator to review?
   c. Will one individual on the management team have the authority to structure and change the terms of an offer?
   d. Once an acquisition deal is signed, do we have in place a step-by-step process, which everyone on the management team knows about, for making the acquisition a success?
   e. Does our management team include an individual skilled in private practice management to oversee the ongoing operation of acquired practices?
   f. Does our hospital have a system in place to "fast-track" administrative support to acquired practices so they can continue to be competitive in the community (for example, purchasing, billing, and so forth)?

for acquiring medical practices is necessary in order to guide acquisition activities and to justify the program if you are ever challenged by your board, your medical staff, or anyone else.

In other words, acquisitions should not occur idly or spontaneously. They must be linked with the hospital's strategic business plan. That plan must precede any acquisition activity in order for the hospital to determine the relationship of practice acquisition to achieving the hospital's overall business objectives. The acquisition game is too risky and too expensive to undertake simply because your closest competitor is doing so.

In all honesty, many hospitals around the country that are buying doctors' practices have not evolved their acquisition programs from their strategic business plans. They have not carefully organized their acquisition efforts to ensure that each purchase fulfills a specific business protection or expansion objective congruent with furthering the hospital's strategies. Some of those efforts have been successful despite the lack of planning. Many of them, however, have resulted in terrible financial failures or have led to medical staff uprisings. This, in turn, can lead to the loss of a job for the hospital administrator and the loss of admissions from former loyalists who were so alienated by the "insensitive" acquisition program that they have become active on a competitor hospital's staff.

The Acquisition Planning Process

A practice acquisition program should be the product of a process in which the hospital's board, medical staff, and management team have all participated. Emphasis must be placed on the word *process* here. The components of that process include both input gathering from and education of the potential participants in the program.

Gathering input from the board, medical staff, and administrative team — and doing so in a very objective, confidential, and well-planned manner — is essential for two reasons. The more obvious reason is to allow each of the parties an opportunity to "buy into" the acquisition process through participation in its development. The less obvious reason is that frequently, during the process of obtaining input, information is gained and resources are identified that become invaluable in pursuing acquisition opportunities once the program moves ahead.

It is not unusual, for example, for a key, actively admitting physician who is being interviewed by a consultant on the subject of acquisition to tell that "outsider" in confidence that he is planning to retire in one or two years and that, before long, he will be interested in discussing the possibility of selling his practice to a hospital. Without having this kind of opportunity to discuss the topic in confidence, most physicians and surgeons are very reluctant to indicate their retirement plans until the last minute, since they do not want the local community to know they are on the verge of leaving their practice. Some hospitals merely survey their doctors to determine if they have an interest in selling their practices to the hospital. These hospitals receive negative responses from some physicians who are not comfortable revealing their plans. This results in the incorrect impression that there is little interest in practice acquisition.

The same input-gathering process provides an opportunity for the management team to educate its board and medical staff as to the acquisition concept and implementation alternatives. In some cases, the mission, culture, and political realities of the hospital are determined not to fit with the concept of practice acquisition. It is common in many situations, however, for board or medical staff concerns about the hospital's owning private practices to dissipate as a result of the input-gathering and educational process, which leads to an understanding of the potential value of acquisition for both the doctors and the hospital.

Although often a surprise for the management team and the board, it is not unusual to discover during the input-gathering process that the majority of the medical staff are not opposed to the concept of acquisition, if undertaken properly. We are all familiar with the saying, "If you never ask, you never find out." Concerns about potentially negative reactions from doctors often hinder administrators from evaluating acquisition as a strategic business development option. Gathering input from the medical staff can not only dissipate those concerns; it can sometimes result in the discovery that many doctors on staff want to know why the hospital has not been more aggressive in pursuing such activities, as has a competitor facility in the same community.

Cultivating Physician Support

No acquisition program should be undertaken by a hospital, including the purchase of even one practice, without first preparing the active medical staff to accept the acquisition. In addition to conducting personal interviews of a cross section of the staff (by specialty, age, activity levels, and so forth) as to their opinions of the concept and their ideas for structuring the program, the entire medical staff should be surveyed by use of a written survey instrument. This alerts all physicians on the staff to the possibility that the hospital may be purchasing doctors' practices and lets them know of the hospital's interest so they might speak with the hospital about the sale of their own practices before going to another hospital.

Due to the potentially controversial nature of acquisition programs at some hospitals, a strategy for the cultivation of physician support should be carefully planned in advance of seeking such support. The written survey on acquisition should not be a surprise to your most important doctors.

Your most loyal, active admitters and other politically important physicians should not suddenly receive a survey in the mail notifying them that the hospital is on the verge of undertaking an acquisition program. Key medical staff leaders should be identified in advance of survey distribution and should be contacted personally and informed of the hospital's intention to gather opinions before making any decision about undertaking such a program. These staff leaders should also be assured that they will be given an early opportunity to provide input for the design of any such program and that no acquisition effort will be undertaken without first considering their preferences.

Although no acquisition program is satisfactory to every doctor on staff, planning the program's specifics with the benefit of input from the doctors will lessen objections to the undertaking. Questions asked of the staff should range from the political and strategic to the operational. For example, the staff should be asked (1) how they feel about the impact of an acquisition program on the medical staff overall; (2) their opinions of the fit of acquisition with the culture of the medical community; and (3) their preferences as to whether practices should be owned by a physician corporation, by the hospital, or by a joint venture corporation.

Corporate Structure

Before undertaking acquisition, the hospital must develop the necessary corporate structure to support acquired practices. Having the proper structure from both the legal and operational standpoints before beginning the acquisition program is invaluable, for you have it in place when you need it in order to respond to an acquisition opportunity. It is unfortunate to see the number of hospitals that have been approached by one of their important physicians and have been invited to buy his or her practice, but that have lost the opportunity and all of the practice's patients to another hospital because they were not ready when the opportunity arose. Your hospital's attorneys should be involved early in the process to advise you (as they did if your hospital went through corporate restructuring) on which for-profit or not-for-profit entity offers the most appropriate home for acquired practices.

How Aggressive Should Your Program Be?

A key decision that should be made as part of practice acquisition planning is whether your hospital is undertaking a reactive or proactive acquisition program. Most often, there are three levels of activity, or degrees of aggressiveness, with which most hospitals pursue acquisition:

1. Reaction to physician-initiated discussions about their desire to sell their practices
2. Notification, usually by mail, to all doctors on the medical staff that the hospital would be interested to hear from any of its physicians who may be considering selling their practices to a hospital
3. Proactive and energetic sales initiatives undertaken by a hospital team to seek out, and successfully win, appropriate acquisition candidates

The first of these levels of activity obviously involves the least visibility for the hospital and usually requires the lowest amount of commitment of both human and financial resources. The second level of activity results in greater visibility by informing the entire medical staff that the hospital is willing to pursue acquisition opportunities. This can lead to a momentary flurry of interest or, perhaps, opposition. This usually dissipates because, in most cases, hospitals choosing this option often communicate only once with their doctors on this topic, and the hospital soon becomes an infrequent participant in acquisition, similar to those choosing the reactive mode.

The third and most aggressive level calls for energetic "go-get-'em" activity, is usually far more costly than the other two, requires continuous activity by senior management, and is most visible to the medical staff and to competitor hospitals. As a result, this level of activity is the one that is most likely to lead, on the one hand, to large-scale controversy and complete termination of the acquisition program or, on the other hand, to the most widespread success, increase in market share, and return on investment for the hospital.

Hospitals choosing one of the first two levels of acquisition activity usually become involved solely with practices that are now active and loyal. The third level of activity calls for the hospital to also go after current medical staff members who split their admissions with another hospital, and to pursue physicians who are not now on that hospital's staff.

The Cost of Acquisition

Undercapitalization has caused some hospital acquisition programs to falter and fail. Hospitals often underestimate the cost of acquisition. Any hospital preparing to pursue this business development strategy should recognize and budget adequately for its two components: Money is needed both to run the acquisition program and to buy the practice from the doctor. If a hospital is serious about an acquisition program, it must be willing to devote significant financial and human resources to pursuing acquisition candidates, to closing the deal, and to maintaining and enhancing those practices on an ongoing basis after the deal is signed.

The possible cost components included in a contract with a physician to buy his or her practice is treated in chapter 7. Let us at this point consider some of the cost elements required for the hospital to run an active acquisition program.

The hospital needs to pay the salary (or portion of a salary) necessary for the manager who is responsible for devoting significant time to overseeing the program and pursuing acquisition candidates. Money is needed for developing materials to use in selling to acquisition candidates in order to impress them with the advantages of affiliation with the hospital. Additional funds are needed by hospitals that choose to use consultants for the technical aspects of acquisition planning, for their involvement with the candidate search process, for the evaluation of candidate practices and for establishing their value, perhaps for their participation in the negotiation process, and for their services to transform acquired practices from private enterprises into hospital satellites. Money is also required to pay lawyers and accountants to orchestrate the financing of the arrangement and to protect the hospital from the many legal pitfalls possible in acquisition activities.

The hospital needs to employ staff who will manage the acquired practices on an ongoing basis and who will act as a liaison between those satellites, the hospital, and its departments. Some portion of the salaries of hospital staff who are employed in human resources, the billing office, planning and marketing, and other departments needs to be apportioned for the time they spend supporting the acquired practices. Additional money is needed for enhancing the practice through computerization, merging with other practices, recruiting additional physicians, launching promotional activities, and so forth.

A hospital acquisition program, whether run under the auspices of the hospital itself or by a separate corporation, deserves its own annual budget in order to succeed. It is not unusual for a hospital that is serious about practice acquisition to spend $500,000 to $1 million or more each year. Some hospitals are realizing as much as a 5 to 1 return on investment. This frequently is the result of new revenues received from practices that formerly had been admitting their patients to other hospitals. But this does not take into account protected hospital revenues resulting from admissions of one of its active physicians that would have been lost to a competitor had the hospital not purchased that physician's practice.

While there can be no contractual requirements for an acquired practice to admit or refer all of its patients to the acquiring hospital, it is natural for the vast majority of them to flow in that direction. Thus, although an acquisition program is costly, a growing number of hospitals find that the return in a successful program can vastly outweigh the cost. They also believe that not undertaking such a program could, in a highly competitive marketplace, result in a tremendous loss of revenue for the hospital. Practice acquisition can therefore be seen to be both an offensive and defensive strategy.

Elements of the Acquisition Plan

When the members of your governing board, medical staff, and senior management have agreed that practice acquisition is an appropriate and potentially valuable strategy to pursue, and when a commitment has been made that the hospital will budget adequate dollars and develop the appropriate organizational structure to support the effort, your next step is to formulate a practical and comprehensive practice acquisition plan. This plan determines the size of the annual acquisition budget and provides specific guidance for organizing and implementing the program. The elements of the acquisition plan are listed in figure 3.2 and described below.

The plan should evolve from a decision as to whether the hospital will undertake a limited and reactive or an aggressive and proactive acquisition process. The elements of the acquisition plan must be driven by their relationship to the objectives of the hospital's strategic business plan. The resulting acquisition plan should provide valuable guidance, while admittedly not always offering black or white answers, as to when the hospital should say yes or no to an acquisition opportunity. The acquisition plan, in other words, should provide *criteria to identify and develop arrangements with appropriate candidates for acquisition.* It can also be helpful to the hospital in turning down a loyal doctor who is interested in selling his or her practice to the hospital.

Figure 3.2. Elements of the Acquisition Plan

1. Objectives of the strategic business plan to be achieved through the acquisition program
2. Total number of practices to be acquired
3. Anticipated schedule for those acquisitions
4. Type and number of acquisitions desired, by specialty
5. Age guidelines
6. Geographic locations targeted
7. Patient-volume goals per practice
8. Payment-mix goals per practice
9. Guidelines for desired number of hospital admissions and referrals per practice
10. Type of specialty referrals desired
11. Ground rules for changing referral patterns of acquired practices
12. Financial expectations from acquired practices and from the acquisition program overall
13. Qualification, quality, and practice-style requirements for physicians under consideration
14. Contractual arrangement and price guidelines for practices to be acquired

In essence, an acquisition plan should set forth the parameters of the acquisition program. This should include a determination of the *desired number of practices* that the hospital intends to acquire in each year of the program. This number should be an outgrowth of the objectives that the hospital wishes to achieve through the program. For example, if a hospital is only implementing an acquisition strategy to protect its current market share, the number of practices to be acquired each year should be based on calculations relating to the number that are needed to maintain the current level of admissions and referrals. Or if a hospital wishes to expand its market share in its primary or secondary service areas or desires to establish a presence in a community that it does not now serve, it needs to determine a different number of acquisitions on the basis of calculations relating to admission goals.

The *timing of acquiring those practices* should be related to the hospital's ability to finance them and to the extent that its human resources are available to implement the program. A hospital new to the acquisition game should proceed slowly in order to ensure the success of the first one or two practices acquired and thereby to enhance the prospects for the hospital's future acquisition plans. For a hospital has much to learn from its first acquisitions, and it will likely make mistakes. Being very aggressive too early with regard to the number of practices pursued can be dangerous to the long-term viability of the program.

The acquisition plan should detail *which practice specialties should be attracted through the program, as well as the number of each.* These decisions are driven by the objectives of the hospital with regard to whether it wishes to expand upon current clinical strengths, fill gaps in clinical areas, build single or multispecialty group practices, develop new product lines, and so forth.

Age guidelines should be included in the acquisition plan as well. Some hospitals prefer only to acquire practices of retiring physicians currently on their staff. Others are interested in acquiring successful practices of physicians of any age so long as they have been out of their residency programs for at least five years. Yet other hospitals are interested in concentrating on practices of younger doctors who have only been in practice for two or three years, because the cost of acquisition is lower and the potential for keeping the doctor involved for a long time and for developing that practice as a multipurpose satellite may be greater.

Geographic location of practices to be acquired should be clearly delineated in the acquisition plan. The reasons for this are both political and strategic. Most hospitals choose to stay away from geographic areas where they would be perceived as being competitive with their current loyal doctors. Strategic reasons for locational analysis and selection include avoiding communities with a payment mix not desired by the hospital or, conversely, going after communities that offer a favorable mix of patients or a great potential for population growth.

Objectives with regard to *patient volumes* desired per practice are also appropriate for inclusion in the acquisition plan. Some hospitals have decided that they will only pursue practices where there is a specified minimum number of active patient records or annual patient visits. Minimum volume expectations for practices can be further complemented by requirements for the *payment mix* within those practices. The hospital may wish to create minimal requirements for insurance coverage of patients within any practice under consideration.

In addition to targets for patient volume and payment mix at the practice, the hospital may wish to establish criteria for *minimum numbers of admissions and referrals* to the hospital that could potentially evolve from a practice. While there are legal constraints on requiring admissions and referrals (see chapter 5), it is reasonable for a hospital to assume that it will receive a fair percentage of cases needing hospitalization from a practice. Those familiar with physician practice patterns are also familiar with, and can apply assumptions regarding, admission and referral volumes that could come from each specialty. This will help the hospital to determine what its reasonable expectations might be from an acquired practice. If the acquisition plan sets forth such criteria, the hospital will have guidance as to whether a practice being considered for acquisition falls within the hospital's targeted volume goals.

The acquisition plan could also incorporate targets as to the *type of specialty referrals* desired from acquired primary care practices. Depending on the objectives of the strategic business plan, the hospital may wish to turn away an opportunity for acquiring a general medical or family practice where the number or type of specialty referrals is different from that desired and is less than what could be forthcoming from another primary care practice.

In their acquisition planning, some hospitals are beginning to incorporate criteria for selecting candidates according to the DRG mix that the hospital prefers. This enables the hospital to be assured that admissions or referrals coming to the hospital will be of the type that the hospital can treat cost-effectively, and for which there are adequate specialists, equipment, and support services available to provide high-quality care.

In their acquisition plans, hospitals should include *ground rules for changing (or not changing) the referral patterns* of acquired practices. Some institutions that have not carefully planned their acquisition programs have required the newly acquired practice to refer all patients to hospital specialists other than those formerly receiving the referrals. Without having fully researched the referral patterns of the practice, those institutions may not know that they are cutting off some specialists currently on their staff who are very important to them. The results are obvious.

The practice acquisition plan should clarify the hospital's *financial expectations* from the acquisition program. Financial expectations for any practice to be considered for acquisition, and expectations of the overall impact of the program on the hospital, should both be determined. This is not to say that financial projections can be made for practices before they are identified, but rather that ground rules should be created in order to satisfy the requirements of the hospital's board and provide guidance to the management team.

A determination should be made of whether each practice must generate a profit for the hospital or whether an adequate outcome of the program would be to have each acquired practice be self-sufficient. Must the acquired practices together generate enough profit to support the cost of the hospital's acquisition program in addition to their own costs? What are the return-on-investment (ROI) goals overall for the hospital's acquisition program? What does everyone agree to as the components of income and expense to be counted in determining ROI? If one practice that has been acquired fails to meet the ROI goals, does the entire program end? These issues should be addressed up front in order to avoid complications later.

Some hospitals choose to incorporate minimum objectives with regard to the *qualifications of physicians* whose practices will be acquired, the *quality-of-care expectations* the hospital has for those practices, *practice-style requirements,* and so forth. The author strongly suggests that any hospital considering acquisition discuss with its current medical staff what the qualifications and quality requirements should be in order to acquire practices that will maintain or enhance the hospital's current level of quality of care and reputation in the community.

A common concern on the part of medical staffs asked by their hospital management team to consider supporting an acquisition program is that the program might result in the purchase of "anything out there" that will bring dollars to the hospital, even at the expense of quality. This concern should be addressed up front and appropriate requirements should be determined for a practice to be considered for acquisition.

Some hospitals, for example, choose to limit their acquisitions to the practices of board-certified physicians. Others only acquire practices of primary care physicians who are willing to participate actively in the care of hospitalized patients. Yet others seek to acquire primary care practices in which the physician wishes to stay out of the hospital and refer all patients to specialists. It is of course sometimes difficult to know whether a set of qualifications such as these is recommended by medical staff members to protect quality or to protect their economic interests. As with many other aspects of the hospital's acquisition program, the hospital's attorneys should be involved from the beginning in carefully reviewing the program to ensure that it does not violate any federal or state laws.

Some hospitals include *guidelines for the contractual arrangements* they will make with acquisition candidates, as well as *limits on the maximum dollar value* of opportunities they will consider. They define, as part of their plan, whether they will only buy practices or will also buy real estate, what formulas they will use for placing a dollar value on practices, and so forth. There are different schools of thought in the industry regarding how detailed an acquisition plan should be with respect to the amount to be paid for an acquired practice. On the one hand, setting standard formulas in advance can help the hospital avoid the appearance of making an overly high offer to a physician not on staff and later angering a very active and loyal physician by making him or her a much lower offer. On the other hand, setting specific guidelines in advance can greatly limit the creativity and flexibility with which the hospital is able to pursue or respond to excellent opportunities.

The Practice Acquisition Team

Once the practice acquisition plan has been completed, you should make sure that the necessary resources are in place to implement the plan effectively. Of primary importance is the availability of the appropriate practice acquisition team with members to perform a variety of roles.

Searching and Selling

An essential role for the practice acquisition team is "searching and selling," that is, searching for appropriate acquisition candidates, selling the opportunity, and helping to bring it to closure. Unfortunately, some hospitals develop an excellent game plan for acquisition and fund it appropriately but do not consider how essential it is to have the "right person" to carry out this function.

The right person is one who has adequate time to devote to the initiative, is very comfortable speaking with physicians and is not intimidated by them, is comfortable assuming responsibility for selling, understands physicians' practices and lifestyles outside the hospital, has the poise and personality to engender respect on the part of the physicians, and so forth. Delegation of this responsibility should not be made solely on the basis of who occupies a particular position.

The chief executive of the hospital may be very conversant with the activities of physicians within the walls of the hospital but may feel limited in his or her knowledge about what goes on within the walls of their private practices. In addition, the time required in the acquisition effort may be far too great for the chief executive to pursue opportunities effectively. Consequently, this role may require someone in a different position who can devote more time.

The vice-president for planning may be the best professional in your state for planning a new hospital building and the services to be included therein, but he or she may not feel comfortable calling on physicians in their private practices to discuss and persuade them to make a major change in their future. The vice-president for marketing may be enormously capable when it comes to new product development or overseeing a major promotional effort but may not be the right person for many physicians to speak with if he or she is perceived as "that person who keeps pushing advertising on us." The medical director of the hospital, depending on his history, may be very well received by physicians but may be viewed as "one of them" and "a doctor who hasn't practiced in many years, so how could he know the realities of the current practice situation?"

Any of these executives (or others, such as the chief financial officer) may be very good or very bad for taking the lead in searching for candidates and selling interest in acquisition. Individual decisions as to the most appropriate person need to be made at each hospital.

There are varied opinions as to the role of a physician in the search for practice candidates. Most hospitals feel that having a doctor involved in relating to other doctors is very valuable. Some hospitals believe, however, that it would be hard to find a physician who would feel comfortable knocking on doors and selling acquisition opportunities to other doctors, or who would be very good at it. When such hospitals consider the doctors on their staff for this role, they often decide that they have some very effective physicians as resources to help close the deal, but that the initial time and effort should be undertaken by a nonphysician who is particularly good at relating to doctors.

Many hospitals decide to fill the search-and-sales role through the use of consulting firms strong in handling the relations between a hospital and its medical staff and that have experience in practice recruitment and acquisition. Those hospitals find it advantageous to use an outside consultant who has the time to make the acquisition program work. Consulting firms are also conversant with private practices, which is appealing to physicians. Initially, it is often easier for physicians to share information about their private practices and their plans for the future with an outsider than with someone who works in the hospital.

Evaluating the Practices

Another important role for the acquisition team is the evaluation of the practices of interested physicians. Whoever is designated to undertake the evaluations must be knowledgeable about all types of doctors' practices and must have solid technical skills in order to analyze the various components of the practice, suggest an appropriate purchase price to the hospital's senior management, and so forth. The "how-to's" of evaluating practices are covered in chapter 6.

Negotiating

Yet another role for the acquisition team is negotiating. Closing on an acquisition opportunity requires many of the same negotiating skills necessary to buy or sell any new business venture. Closing also requires knowledge of doctors' practices and the ability to command respect from, and relate to, physicians. In addition, it requires the authority to speak for the hospital. Most often, the chief executive officer fills this role. In some cases, responsibility for closing is assigned to the executive vice-president, chief financial officer, or some other member of the senior management staff.

As with the activity involved in searching for and approaching candidates, as well as with conducting technical evaluations of practices being considered, some hospitals choose to involve consultants in the negotiation process. Although consultants are not usually the primary negotiators, their membership on the team can be helpful if they have already established some basis of trust with the physicians.

Whether the chief negotiator teams up with another member of the hospital's management team or with a consultant, the two can function as a "dynamic duo" and can play different roles in helping the physician consider the opportunity. Either one can play the primary role as the negotiator, or he or she can play the role of the physician's most amenable contact. Whoever plays the primary negotiating role must have skills in developing creative arrangements and negotiating and must have the authority to close.

Managing the Practice

Still another function of the acquisition team is the ongoing management of the practice after it has been acquired. This requires both the ability to relate well to physicians and their office staffs and knowledge of, if not experience in, practice management. As is discussed in the final chapter of this book, a great mistake made by some hospitals that have successfully acquired practices is that they fail to develop a streamlined process for on-going administrative support of the practice after the deal is negotiated. They require acquired practices to go through the hospital's usual administrative departments for support services. The resulting confusion, slowdown in operations, and frustration for the doctor, his or her office staff, and patients has more than once led to the divorce of a practice from its acquiring hospital soon after the papers were signed. Hence the hospital must identify a qualified person to oversee the support activities for acquired practices on an ongoing basis.

It would be nearly impossible for any one person to be good at all of the roles necessary to run an effective hospital acquisition program. Usually, two or three senior managers are needed to make the process work. Whatever the size and composition of the team, a team leader should be identified at the outset. This should be a member of the team who has been given the major responsibility for, and a significant amount of time to devote to, making the acquisition process work.

Identifying Acquisition Candidates

Your hospital is now ready to develop a list of physicians to approach to explore their interest in selling their practices. Each of the candidates must fit with the goals and criteria identified in the acquisition plan. The list of candidates should be reviewed with friendly doctors on your staff to pre-qualify each name to the extent possible and to eliminate those who do not fit the criteria set forth in the plan. Not all names on the list will be known to your physician advisers. Candidate identification, of course, presumes that your hospital has decided to undertake a proactive search for practices.

List of Potential Candidates

The first step is to identify a complete list of potential candidates. The sources for such a list are fairly standard across the country, with some local exceptions: Some areas of the country have published directories of medical professionals, which can be valuable sources of information to augment the other resources available for the identification of physicians practicing in any geographic area. In the Philadelphia area, for example, you can purchase a directory of physicians that includes information on hospital affiliation, the medical school and residency program from which the physician has graduated, and so forth. No one directory is complete or totally accurate. A nearly complete list seems to result only from an evaluation of all of the directories available.

Standard resources listing physicians practicing in any geographic area, which can be used to identify candidates for acquisition, usually include the following:

- *Telephone directories.* Throughout the United States the "Yellow Pages" are probably the most commonly used source for physicians' names. While helpful, they are also very limited in that information is generally restricted to the physician's name, the office address, the telephone number, and sometimes the specialty. More information may be available if the physician has purchased a display advertisement.
- *Medical society and specialty society directories.* Whether national, state, or local, these directories often provide valuable information on physicians beyond what may be found in the telephone book. The problem with these directories is that some of them do not delineate

physicians according to a small enough geographic area to be practical without also referring to the local telephone directory. Use of such directories, where physicians are listed alphabetically by state, can be an exhausting and expensive procedure for candidate identification. Directories that provide a breakdown of physician names by small geographic area are of greatest value for the search.

- *Hospital medical staff directories.* Few sources are as valuable as the medical staff listings of your competitor hospitals. This is especially true if they have developed more than a simple listing of their medical staff, namely a referral directory or consultant's directory for use by their physicians. Such directories provide valuable information on group practice membership, specialties and subspecialties of physicians, office locations, perhaps board certification, and so forth.

    It is surprising how many hospitals do not feel that they can obtain their competitor's medical staff directories. Nevertheless, any good hospital market research initiative requires having information about the competitor hospital's physicians. A little creativity and ingenuity can give rise to such directories. They are easily obtained by identifying physicians on your own staff who are friends of your hospital and who have multiple staff appointments. Ask them if they would get you a medical staff directory of other hospitals where they have appointments.

Once all of the directories have been gathered, you can begin to build your candidate list. Using your practice acquisition plan for guidance, pursue all of the names in the directories to determine which ones are in accord with the criteria set forth in the plan. For example, physicians whose office locations are outside the targeted areas identified in the acquisition plan obviously should not be considered; those whose office locations are within the targeted areas should be eliminated if they do not meet the specialty requirements of the plan; and so forth.

While age is not listed in most directories, a careful review of the date of a physician's medical school or residency program graduation can often be an indication of approximate age. This can result in further elimination of names from the field when the acquisition plan calls for candidates to be within a certain age range. Or if an objective of the plan is to attract general practitioners only, a careful review of the directories can reveal the general internists who are also active in a subspecialty of internal medicine and, therefore, unlikely to be appropriate candidates.

This approach presumes that the acquiring hospital is interested both in the practices of physicians on its own medical staff and in those physicians not on its staff. The reader is urged not to eliminate from the list the names of physicians who are currently on the hospital's medical staff but who have historically sent very few patients to the hospital (in favor of maintaining an active medical staff affiliation with a competitor). Many hospitals make the mistake of thinking that because a doctor has not sent them many patients over the years, there would be no interest on the part of the physician in selling his or her practice to the hospital. This is often not the case. All physicians meeting the plan's criteria should be approached, whether or not they have been active at the hospital.

Extensive research, such as that mentioned in the preceding sections, is advisable in order to create the most comprehensive and relevant target list possible. This will greatly reduce the amount of time and money spent on pursuing unqualified or inappropriate candidates and will result in the development of an extremely valuable information profile on the qualified candidates who will be approached.

Medical Staff Review of Candidates

The second step in the identification of acquisition candidates is to decide which of your medical staff members should review the list of candidates in order to determine whether the doctors remaining on the list are appropriate and desirable candidates. The decision is both political and practical. You do not want to approach physicians who are not loyal to your hospital, for the very next day they may be alerting your competitor hospital or communicating with the targeted candidates to sour them on your institution. In addition, you should avoid physicians who are loyal but who are known to be indiscreet about sharing information.

From a practical standpoint, you should approach physicians who you think are most likely to know the candidates on the list. Consequently, the chief of internal medicine should be approached regarding internists, the chief of family practice with regard to family practitioners, and so forth. Do not overlook the value of approaching your specialists for their knowledge of primary care physicians, since it is very possible that your specialists may know such doctors well as the result of receiving referrals from them. If your hospital has a policy of entering the names of all referring or family physicians on your hospital's patient admitting form, you have invaluable data for identifying specialists on your staff who are sources of information about primary care physicians not on your staff (or who are relatively inactive at the hospital).

When reviewing the list of candidates with your physician advisers, you should pursue your leads thoroughly. For example, if your chief of medicine tells you he knows one of the listed doctors only slightly but is aware that he is very active at a particular golf club, or is friendly with one of the other doctors on your staff, or is a member of a particular church or synagogue, approach the candidate's friend or another loyal doctor on your staff who is involved in the same organization to explore their knowledge of the candidate further. This often leads to rich rewards when the time comes to attempt a practice acquisition.

In addition, be sure to review the candidates' names with your politically important medical staff leaders. It is essential to avoid having the president of the medical staff announce at a meeting of the board of trustees that he has not been consulted about the program and therefore does not feel comfortable with it, and that he has heard the hospital is cultivating a physician whose reputation for quality is highly questionable. This scenario is all too common and can lead to a rapid deterioration of the administration's credibility and to the discontinuation of the acquisition effort.

Approaching Acquisition Candidates

The first step in the pursuit of candidates is to obtain a personal meeting with them. No attempt should be made to fully present the idea of acquisition over the telephone or in writing. Valuable opportunities have been lost during the first telephone or letter contact by hospital representatives seeking to establish serious interest on the part of physicians before meeting with them. The likelihood of the concepts being adequately presented, and the physicians' concerns being satisfactorily addressed, are far greater if the issues are discussed in person (either at the physician's office or at another location outside the hospital). Hence the primary goal is to obtain the first meeting.

The First Meeting

It sounds much simpler than it often is to obtain the first meeting with an acquisition candidate. Unless you have a personal friend of the candidate available to set up the meeting for you, you must make a decision as to whether to approach the physician for a first meeting by letter or by telephone. Both can work. The key with either approach is to present just enough information to arouse interest and curiosity, but not so much as to give the physician a reason to say no.

Both the letter and the telephone call must first go through the physician's office staff. Getting through to the doctor may not be easy, depending on his or her administrative style and that of the office staff. Careful consideration should be given in advance to the exact content of the written or telephone message. One of the most successful approaches is to indicate that you "would like to tell Dr. X about opportunities and support programs the hospital has been making available to area physicians and which have been of great interest to them."

There is always a danger, as a result of the first contact, that a doctor will run to another hospital's CEO, even though this doctor has scheduled a meeting with you. Some doctors do this in order to let the hospital where they are more active know what is going on and thus avoid being considered disloyal if word about the meeting gets out. Yet others do this to "suggest" to the other hospital that they may lose an active practice if they cannot come up with a better offer.

You must also consider how to conduct the conversation once you are in the door for the first meeting. You, or the hospital representative approaching the physician, must have good intuitive abilities to determine whether a direct or indirect approach is more appropriate for the personality across the table from you. Some physicians prefer that you come right to the point, and they will respect you for doing so. They feel they have been generous in giving you a half-hour of their time. They are aware that their patient waiting room is full and that the telephone is ringing for them. They do not appreciate "public relations visits" in the middle of their workday. For this reason, some hospitals believe that visits to physicians' offices should only be made early in the morning, in the evening, or on weekends. Realistically, though, many physicians are unwilling to spend their nights or weekends having such conversations until they are really interested in the concept. They will require that you meet them during the workweek.

Other physicians are more comfortable with a roundabout rather than direct approach. This is not to suggest that you should in any way mislead the physicians with whom you are speaking. To do so would result in turning off any high-quality physician you may wish to attract. What is being suggested, rather, is that the opportunity be taken (especially with physicians who are not familiar with your hospital) to impress them about the hospital and its relationship with its doctors by first telling them about the hospital's physician-support programs. You should tell them how the hospital has been helping to maximize the practice success of its active, loyal physicians through a variety of medical staff initiatives. This will perhaps impress the candidate with the fact that your hospital is doing far more for its physicians than the hospital where the doctor is currently affiliated.

You should also take the opportunity to identify briefly some of the more impressive and sophisticated services available at your hospital. You may wish to highlight a few strengths of your hospital that may be sources of frustration for him and his patients at his own hospital. Having researched such information about your competitors will give you the opportunity to put your own hospital in the best light. Obviously, if the candidate is currently on your staff and actively uses your hospital, much of this information will not be necessary, and a more direct approach may be used sooner.

It is essential during the course of the conversation that you look for a hook with which to further evoke the physician candidate's interest in selling his practice to the hospital. Hospital management professionals have not historically viewed themselves as salesmen, and they may be offended by the concept of selling and thinking in terms such as *hook*. Such words are more commonly understood to be used by realtors, automobile dealers, computer system salesmen, and so forth. The fact is, however, that hospitals wishing to succeed at acquisition in a highly competitive environment must sell. If the hospital representative approaching physician candidates is not comfortable with this technique, he or she is the wrong person for the job.

Selling hospital acquisition opportunities is not the same as selling automobiles. The approach must be sophisticated, quality oriented, and sincere. No marriage between a physician's private practice and a hospital will work over the long term if this is not the case. However, a professional, somewhat "laid-back" sales effort is essential for the initiative to succeed. Hence the hospital representative must look for a hook.

If the physician has an interest, it will often appear in some indirect way. You must be adept enough at interviewing people to pick up this hint of interest. The physician candidate may be unaware that he could have an interest in selling his practice to the hospital and is not hinting at such interest purposely. He is just not yet ready to recognize the possible advantages of the idea. Therefore, you must seek out the physician's need that could be filled through acquisition and cultivate discussion about it.

One example might be as apparent as a physician's statement that he or she will be considering retirement in a year or two. Less obvious is a statement of frustration with one or more aspects of the doctor's current hospital affiliation. Or perhaps he or she gives an indication of increasing annoyance with the amount of time required to manage the business side of private practice. Each of these statements offers an opportunity for the hospital representative to pursue. Following further discussion, it may soon become apparent to a physician that her interest in retiring, or her frustration with her current hospital affiliation, or her desire to relieve herself of administrative responsibilities represents enough of a reason to cause her to explore (on a very preliminary basis) the sale of her practice to your hospital.

The Hospital Visit

The next step in the acquisition process is to encourage the physician to visit your hospital. Even doctors who have been practicing at your hospital for years usually appreciate an invitation to the president's office for a meeting to discuss the future plans of the hospital in relation to the physician's future plans. If a candidate has never been active at or stepped foot inside the hospital, you should invite him for a tour of the facility and a meeting with the leadership of the institution.

Before the candidate visits the hospital, be sure to prepare the hospital team to receive and impress him. Many aspects of this visit can be likened to the process that a hospital undertakes to successfully recruit a new doctor to town. A team should be identified and prepared to fulfill a variety of objectives, including presenting the advantages of affiliation with the hospital.

Team members could include the chairman and possibly other physicians from the candidate's potential clinical department, an elected medical staff leader, a nursing leader, the CEO, and any other appropriate senior hospital manager. So as not to overwhelm the physician or require too much time, the first visit may actually only allow for a meeting with the CEO and perhaps one physician. The rest of the team's activity could be scheduled for a subsequent visit. Nevertheless, roles need to be identified up front, questions must be answered, and the team must be ready for the candidate's arrival.

During this visit, the CEO (or whoever has been identified as the primary negotiator) and the candidate should try to get to know each other and should be very direct with one another. The candidate has already made time available in his or her office for the first meeting and has devoted more time to come to the hospital for a second meeting. He or she will not be willing to spend even more time unless the opportunity is discussed in some detail and the CEO is willing to be very straightforward about the possible advantages and disadvantages of affiliation with the hospital. In order to conduct this session, the CEO and his or her advisers need to have prepared carefully and determined the approximate parameters of the acquisition arrangement.

No offer should be made on the first visit of the candidate physician to the hospital. The hospital does not yet know enough about the doctor's practice to make an offer covering dollar amounts or the specifics of the arrangement. No detailed evaluation of the physician's practice has yet been undertaken. Most doctors do not feel comfortable allowing a comprehensive evaluation of their practice to occur (especially of finances) until after they have had some discussion with the chief executive of the acquiring hospital and have determined whether they might have a serious interest in the opportunity.

At this meeting, however, many of the options can be discussed. The doctor can learn more about the practical realities of selling his or her practice to the hospital. Examples can be presented of alternative arrangements that the hospital might be willing to consider. The hospital can further describe business support services it has available for acquired practices, and so forth.

In addition, you must make sure that the discussion covers *the* frustration, concern, or interest that the physician identified during the first visit to his office as the basis for his possible willingness to consider an acquisition opportunity. If it is obtaining liquidity out of his practice before retirement, gaining long-term security for his family, relieving himself of the headaches of administering the practice, or whatever, this must be discussed at the meeting. Only then can the hospital understand and respond to the physician's greatest area of interest so that the doctor leaves the meeting having more fully recognized the real benefits of affiliation. He may then be willing to discuss the acquisition further.

Telephone Follow-up

Unless the physician indicates his willingness to go further with the opportunity before ending his visit, interest is usually determined by a telephone call from the physician to the CEO after the meeting. Some hospitals find it desirable not to wait for the physician to call the CEO. Rather, several days after the hospital visit, the CEO calls the physician to help him consider the opportunity. This call is not for the purpose of asking him whether he has decided to sell his practice to the hospital. It is instead for the purpose of telling him that no decision on selling is expected now and of inquiring whether further discussion would be helpful to him in determining if he wishes to have his practice evaluated. Often, helping the candidate to consider the opportunity after the hospital visit causes him to feel comfortable enough to go to the next step, a detailed acquisition evaluation.

Before examining the how-to's of evaluating a practice for acquisition, the following two chapters consider the structural models and legal issues relating to acquisition arrangements and similar initiatives.

Chapter 4

Structuring the Relationship

Ross E. Stromberg

Just as there can be myriad objectives behind a hospital-physician bonding transaction, there are also many ways to structure the relationship. The objective may be as simple as responding to a solo practitioner who wishes to sell his or her practice or as complex as developing a strategy in which the hospital and many of its key physician leaders wish to establish a number of primary care centers on a joint venture basis, with the ambitious goal of locking up their regional marketplace. Each transaction calls for a structure specifically tailored to its unique circumstances and to the goals and concerns of its potential participants.

Thus a critical first step is to have a clear understanding of the circumstances and the key objectives and issues of those who will be affected. Often this includes not only the physicians directly involved but others who may be indirectly affected by the transaction or will likely have viewpoints that the hospital and other project sponsors should take into account as they proceed. For example, if a hospital acquires a practice, will this transaction establish a precedent for future practices offered for sale? How will other members of the medical staff react to a hospital's sponsoring the development of primary care centers by itself or with an existing multispecialty group practice or a small group of key physician leaders? Is it necessary or desirable to open such programs on a broader basis to other physicians? Even if certain key physicians are not interested in selling their practices or investing in a primary care center strategy, should the hospital allow such physicians to participate in the decision-making process and, if so, how?

Hospital managers must keep in mind that the physician's opportunity to participate in the decision-making process may be more important than participation in the venture itself. Human nature being what it is, many physicians who perceive themselves to be frozen out of the transaction will oppose it; but if their viewpoint can be heard within the development phase or if they are given an opportunity to invest in the transaction, they may stop opposing the project and become neutral or even supportive even if they do not subsequently invest in the project.

Once the chief facts are known and the decision makers have identified the likely participants as well as their major goals and concerns, hospital managers can begin examining the various structures of physician-hospital bonding, with the view of developing a lasting relationship that is satisfactory to all participants on a clinical and economic basis. The goal is to create a certain professional and economic interdependence in which both the hospital and the physicians view that relationship to be stronger than their own self-interest.

Alternative Arrangements Other Than Practice Acquisition

Some strategies can satisfy the objectives of physician-hospital bonding without the participants' having to transfer ownership of practices. These strategies include (1) administrative support services and (2) clinical support services.

Administrative Support Services for Physician Practices

A hospital can support the administration of physician practices in several ways:

- *Group purchasing of supplies for individual practitioners.* With the hospital's assistance, the economic benefit of volume purchasing can be passed on to physician participants. However, there are limits to a not-for-profit hospital's making available to physicians supplies it has purchased by reason of its not-for-profit status.[1]
- *Drug repackaging.*
- *Computer networking.* Hospitals can furnish computer hardware to participating physicians that links individual physician terminals with the hospital system, thereby allowing physicians to track patients in the hospital and easing medical record keeping. Health care providers are only scratching the surface of being able to link satellite offices to central practice settings such as multispecialty group practices or the hospital itself, in terms of both clinical and business operational data.
- *Strategic planning and marketing for individual physician practices.* Both physicians and hospitals are justifiably concerned about where the next patient is coming from, and the hospital is uniquely qual-

ified to offer physicians an array of strategic planning and marketing services.

- *Professional liability insurance.* While the details of this strategy are beyond the scope of this book, hospitals should be aware that a number of imaginative approaches are available to tailor professional liability coverage programs for their medical staff members, especially as a result of the 1986 amendments to the federal Risk Retention Act.[2] Each hospital and its physicians have the unique ability to design an effective risk management program that has the potential to be translated into significant savings in the cost of a malpractice insurance program. Whether this program is designed as a volume purchase of insurance from existing carriers or captives (risk-purchasing group), as a risk retention group, or as a self-insurance program, it has the potential to achieve demonstrable savings over existing liability insurance programs. Compared to other practice enhancement arrangements with less economic return to physicians, such programs can result in a true bonding of physicians to the hospital.

The preceding list only highlights the wide spectrum of management and administrative support services that might be offered to physicians either as a complete managed practice or on a menu basis. No matter which services are eventually used, participating physicians do not legally change the structure of their practice. Any one or more of these services are provided by the hospital or its affiliates through contracts to participating physicians who continue to retain the legal ownership of their practice.

Clinical Support Services for Physician Practices

Clinical support services more directly address the clinical aspects of a physician's practice than do hospital services that support the administration of a practice. However, as with administrative support services, clinical support services generally involve a contractual relationship between the hospital and the physicians in which the physicians retain ownership of their existing practices. Examples include:

- *Selective contracting assistance.* Physicians, like hospitals, are often flooded with proposals for contracts from health maintenance organizations (HMOs), preferred provider organizations (PPOs), and insurance companies. As individual practitioners, physicians often feel overwhelmed by such proposals, each with its unique characteristics, including payment mechanisms and other terms and conditions to be met. The hospital, generally in cooperation with interested physicians, has an opportunity to establish a service to analyze such proposals on the basis of predetermined guidelines and to provide summaries to the physicians whereby they can make a more informed judgment.

- *Joint ventures.* Single purpose joint ventures such as imaging centers have the potential to enhance the clinical aspects of physicians' practices while at the same time creating an economic interdependence between the hospital and physicians through shared investment.
- *Joint risk taking through managed care programs.* Managed care programs can take a variety of forms, ranging from "plain vanilla" PPOs to fully capitated HMOs. These programs also include direct contract approaches to the self-insured employer by hospitals and physicians on a cooperative basis. The relationship of physicians and hospitals in managed care programs can be totally independent or can represent a significant sharing of interest and risk, as in mutual contracts or even joint venture ownership of the managed care programs. Regardless of the legal structure of a managed care program or the legal relationship of the hospital and physician to the program, the more the program attracts patients and revenue to the hospital and physician, the stronger the economic interdependence between the providers will be.
- *Medical consultancies and directorships.* This category of services covers a number of different arrangements. Examples include the appointment of a physician as a consultant or medical director of a new clinical program in the institution, such as chemical dependency, in vitro fertilization, or AIDS control. The creation of a clinical institute or "center of excellence" combining dedicated clinical services, research, and fund development can also lead to the creation of one or more medical directorships. These arrangements are contractual in that the physician serves either as a hospital employee or as an independent contractor. Such arrangements can also involve only clinical responsibilities (such as supervising physician services) or only administrative responsibilities (such as supervising nonclinical personnel) or both. The physician can be hired on a part-time or full-time basis, and compensation for services rendered can be by salary or stipend and can be fixed or be tied to some floating economic measure such as the gross operational revenue of the program. If the physician assumes a medical directorship on a full-time basis, the relationship may also have to address the disposition of his or her pre-existing practice, including the possibility of its acquisition by the hospital or an affiliate of the hospital.

This category has significant promise in its application to multiple physician opportunities, particularly given its flexibility, the ability to combine this approach with other practice enhancement strategies, and its traditional characteristics when compared to practice acquisition. It predictably will take on increased use as a potential hospital-physician bonding technique.

Practice Acquisition Strategies

The acquisition of physician practices can be approached in an almost infinite number of ways structurally, but the following list sets forth the key strategies:

- The hospital assists a legally independent physician group in its acquisition of practices.
- The hospital acquires the nonclinical aspects of a practice and leases them back to the practitioner.
- The hospital acquires both clinical and nonclinical aspects of the practice.
- A joint venture is formed between the hospital and physicians to develop physician practices.

Each of these strategies and their alternatives are discussed in the pages that follow.[3]

Assisting a Legally Independent Physician Group in Its Acquisition of Practices

In one strategy, an existing single specialty or multispecialty group practice approaches the hospital for assistance in developing a series of satellites through practice acquisitions (figure 4.1). The satellites, which probably become part of a professional corporation, are staffed by owner-physicians, employed physicians, and/or independent contracting physicians.

Figure 4.1. Model for Hospital-Assisted Expansion of an Independent Physician Group

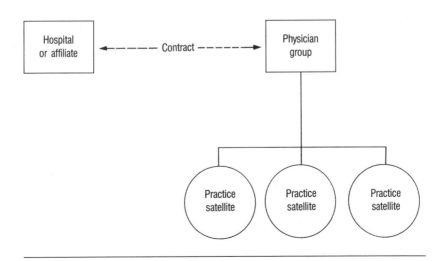

An alternative to this strategy may be several physicians desiring to start up a fully integrated group by combining their practices and acquiring other practices. Again, the resulting structure is probably a professional corporation, and the hospital may be requested to perform a supportive role.

In either arrangement, the hospital's role may include any of the following services:

- Serving as a neutral facilitator.
- Offering strategic planning assistance in formulating the overall strategy of the group practice and determining how this strategy relates to the hospital and its own strategies.
- Providing initial seed capital for the planning function.
- Providing more extensive capital in the strategy's implementation phase. This may include loans, start-up capital, and/or guarantee of debt (in whole or part).
- Providing facilities such as satellite practice sites. This could include using existing hospital properties, upgrading facilities, equipping and leasing such sites to the physician group, purchasing or leasing new sites, and/or making such sites available to the physician group through sale, lease, or other forms of use arrangement. The development of such sites can be by the hospital alone or on a joint venture basis with the group practice and/or other investors such as real estate developers or local investors in the areas to be served by the satellite center.
- Providing administrative support services to the group practice, such as personnel, billing and collection, computer linkage, and marketing services.
- Providing full management of the practice pursuant to a management agreement.

Any one or all such services can be furnished by the hospital or by an affiliated entity.

Key operational issues for this strategy include:

- How to minimize concern by nonparticipating physicians that the hospital is showing favoritism toward the group practice.
- How to ensure that the group practice is responsive to the hospital in terms of the group practice's use of hospital facilities and services, patient referrals, and the like. The key here is creating an effective working relationship between the hospital and the group practice, resulting in a mutually acceptable economic interdependence.
- How to ensure that the hospital's commitment is finite in terms of aggregate dollars and time. Can either party terminate the relationship? If so, what are the consequences for the hospital in terms of its economic commitment to the project?

- How effectively and efficiently the hospital can manage private office practices and provide related administrative support services.
- Whether to compensate the hospital on a fixed fee basis or on a floating basis, such as percentage of gross revenues from the group practice.

Key legal issues for this strategy include:

- Private inurement in terms of avoiding "giving away the farm" to the medical group practice.
- Antifraud and abuse implications of mandating referrals from the group practice to the hospital. In addition, comparable concerns may exist under state medical practice acts.

These legal issues are discussed in chapter 5.

Once this assisting arrangement is established, it may serve as a springboard for further integration, such as joint ventures or managed care risk-taking opportunities. It may even evolve into greater integration of legal ownership between the group practice and the hospital.

Acquiring the Nonclinical Aspects of a Practice and Leasing Them Back to the Practitioner

Not infrequently, hospitals are presented with a proposal to purchase the nonclinical aspects of a practice and lease them back to the practitioner. For example, a physician who is an important user of hospital services may wish to be relieved from the administrative aspects of his or her practice and proposes to the hospital that it assume his or her lease (or buy a building) and take over the day-to-day management of the practice, allowing the physician to concentrate on the practice of medicine. The physician does not want to sell the practice per se but only the aspects that are nonclinical.

Another example is where a key admitter is slowing down his or her practice. In this case, the hospital wants to assist in the orderly transition of the practice to other physicians.

The physicians in both examples can be served by the sale/lease-back model, in which only selected assets and liabilities are transferred to the hospital (figure 4.2). The practitioner retains the clinical aspects as well as the legal form of the practice, whether he or she is a solo practitioner, a partnership, or a professional corporation.

The sale/lease-back model may involve the purchase and/or transfer to the hospital of:

- The physician's facility (ownership of a building or the physician's leasehold interest in a building owned by others)
- Equipment

Figure 4.2. Sale/Lease-Back Model for Hospital Acquisition of Nonclinical Aspects of a Practice

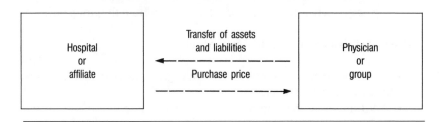

- Personnel
- Supplies and inventory

Accounts receivable and patients' records are generally retained by the practitioner.

Once transferred, such assets may be leased back to the physician, along with a management and administrative services agreement in which the hospital is compensated for services rendered. These assets and services will most likely be augmented by additional services such as strategic planning and marketing and the joint pursuit of managed care opportunities. A variation of this model is where the facilities are not leased back but are otherwise disposed of, and the practitioner relocates his or her practice to another practice setting arranged for by the hospital.

The sale/lease-back model may involve only a single practitioner, or it could involve a number of individual practitioners, with each likely to have an ad hoc arrangement because of the variety of practice settings to be transferred and leased back. In addition, this model is applicable to a transaction involving a larger group practice that has similar objectives, that is, to retain the medical practice but transfer the nonclinical aspects to the hospital. Whereas the magnitude of this type of transaction is greater, the structure remains the same: transfer of selected, nonclinical aspects of the practice and retention by the group practice of its legal structure and clinical aspects.

Key operational issues for this strategy include:

- Whether the practitioner is going to continue in practice indefinitely, or whether a transition arrangement must be made almost immediately
- How the value of the assets and liabilities are to be transferred, and how to reach an amicable agreement with the practitioner on what this value is

- How to prevent the practitioner from going on "cruise control"
- How to avoid becoming a repository for bad real estate deals and failing practices
- How to fit practitioners into broader hospital strategies where the physician practices remain independent
- Whether the hospital can manage a private practice, which is considerably different from acute care services

Key legal issues for this strategy include:

- Private inurement.
- Antifraud and abuse (for example, mandated referrals).
- Due diligence: the hospital must understand fully what it is buying (liabilities as well as assets) and must eliminate any surprises (see chapter 5).

Acquiring Both Clinical and Nonclinical Aspects of a Practice

The acquisition of both clinical and nonclinical aspects of a practice involves the cessation by the practitioner of his or her current legal structure and the beginning of practice in a new legal setting. This setting can be as:

- A physician employee of the hospital or its affiliate, or
- An independent contractor beginning a new practice

Both of these alternatives are described as a single-tiered approach (see figure 4.3). Another alternative is for the physician to become a new member of a hospital-related group practice; this is described as a two-tiered approach (see figure 4.4). The transaction could involve a single practitioner or a number of individual practitioners, each with ad hoc transfer arrangements; or the transaction could be the acquisition of a physician group that wishes to transfer both the clinical and nonclinical aspects of its practice. The new configuration may evolve further into a large, complex arrangement with multiple sites and centralized management services. A salient feature distinguishing these approaches from the joint venture approach (to be discussed later) is that, for all practical purposes, the hospital or its controlled affiliate owns and operates the entire practice.

Once the practice is acquired, it is operated either as a hospital outpatient department or as a new, private office practice. In the single-tiered approach, the hospital exercises considerable control in that the physician has sold and transferred his or her entire practice and becomes a professional employee of the hospital (or its affiliate) or provides services in the new practice setting as an independent contractor. Factors that help determine

Figure 4.3. Single-Tiered Approach to Acquisition of Physician Practices

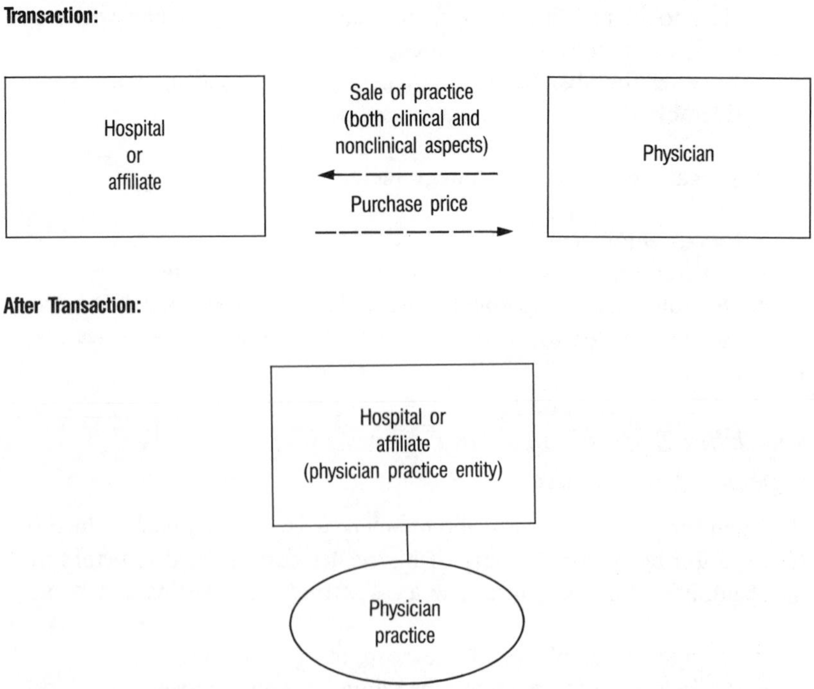

Transaction:

After Transaction:

whether a physician becomes an employee or an independent contractor include corporate practice of medicine considerations (as discussed in chapter 5), the political acceptability of one choice over the other, and the desirability of fringe benefits associated with employment, such as the availability of professional liability insurance and participation in the hospital's pension plan.

The two-tiered approach also involves the complete sale and transfer of a practice but bifurcates the nonclinical from the clinical aspects of the practice, with the former going to the hospital or its affiliate, described as the ambulatory services organization (ASO), and the latter to a related group practice (RGP).

The ASO furnishes, on a turnkey basis, all facilities and services required by the RGP. In addition, the ASO may contract with managed care programs and subcontract with the RGP for physician services. The ASO may also furnish management and administrative services to unrelated physicians.

Figure 4.4.   Two-Tiered Approach to Acquisition of Physician Practices

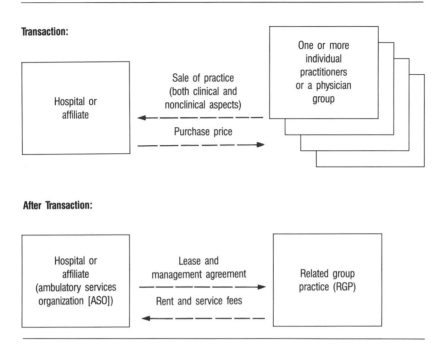

Hospitals have a number of options for structuring the ASO. First, it may be operated as a division of the hospital. Second, it may be operated as a division of the parent holding company. Third, it may be operated as a division of the hospital affiliate, where the ASO can be either a tax-exempt or taxable subsidiary of the hospital or the parent holding company.

The RGP can be a preexisting, legally independent, single or multispecialty group practice, or it can be "related" legally to the hospital. The latter could take a variety of forms: First, the RGP could be a professional corporation wholly owned by a single practitioner-shareholder who also serves as the medical director of the hospital or ASO or is otherwise closely identified with the hospital and its objectives. Second, the RGP could be owned in part by physicians closely tied to the hospital, such as primary care physicians and/or key specialists benefiting from primary care referrals developed through the RGP. Third, the owner-physicians could be practitioners nominated for ownership by the executive committee of the medical staff. Fourth, the physicians who practice as employees of the RGP can be its shareholder-owners. Or fifth, the RGP could be structured as some combination of these alternatives.

While the hospital cannot own equity in a professional corporation, it may have significant practical influence over the RGP. Factors of influence include (1) the RGP's reliance on the hospital for facilities and management and administrative services pursuant to a turnkey contractual arrangement; (2) medical direction furnished to the RGP by the hospital through the ASO; (3) managed care contract opportunities furnished by the hospital; and (4) the practical ability to influence shareholder status in the RGP. The key here is not legal control but, rather, the creation of a mutually satisfactory working relationship in which the economic interdependence of the parties is significant and the commitment of the parties to the retention and expansion of that interdependence is more important than economic self-interest.

Figure 4.5 illustrates a hospital system that has developed a primary care strategy involving the ownership and operation of multiple sites and that arranges for physician services through a number of independent contracts. No separate group-practice entity was formed; rather, attributes of group practice are addressed through less formal policies and procedures:

Figure 4.5. Sample Primary Care Strategy Involving Acquisition of Clinical and Nonclinical Aspects of Physician Practices

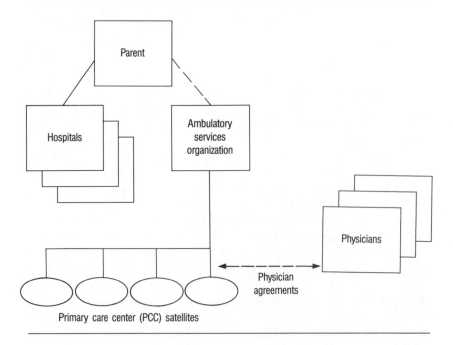

- Primary care center (PCC) satellites are staffed by individual physicians who are ASO employees or who are independent contractors. In either case, these physicians practice full-time in the satellites. Their compensation can have incentives similar to those found in group practices, for example, some risk sharing. Also, although a legal group is not formed, professional collegiality or comparable attributes of group practices can be developed.
- Back-up specialty coverage is ensured through contracts with designated subspecialty groups.
- The medical director establishes clinical practices and procedures.
- The ASO may commit its satellites and participating physicians to managed care opportunities.
- The ASO may furnish management and administrative services to unrelated physicians.

From a hospital system standpoint, this model has the advantage of greater system influence given the absence of an organized group of physicians, which the system fears may otherwise "turn around and bite." However, the disadvantage is that this model may not be accepted by physicians in many situations.

Key operational issues for the acquisition of both clinical and nonclinical aspects of a practice include:

- How to value the practice.
- How to prevent the physician from going on "cruise control."
- How to avoid purchasing practices as a precedent. That is, the purchase of one practice should not establish a precedent, putting pressure on the hospital to buy other practices.
- How to gain physician acceptance of the program.

The key legal issues include, in essence, all of the issues discussed in chapter 5.

Forming a Joint Venture between the Hospital and the Physician Practice

Joint venturing is similar to the two-tiered approach of figure 4.4 in that it involves the transfer of both clinical and nonclinical aspects of practices, the cessation of the selling physician's current legal structure, and the replacement thereof by a new practice setting. Joint venturing differs from the two-tiered approach in that it involves the joint ownership of the practice structure by the hospital and the participating physicians. Given this added element, joint venturing should probably be used only in multiple practice transactions where the overall scope of the strategy can support the added organizational complexity.

This strategy can be framed with a number of variables and, as such, can best be illustrated by an example: A medical center has been approached by several primary care physicians independently exploring the sale of their practices to the hospital. Some specialists have recently raised some concerns about the need to expand the primary care referral base both in the medical center's secondary service area as well as in its primary service area. The medical center has operated several urgent care centers with mixed results and with a strong adverse reaction from members of its medical staff, which have vocally challenged the hospital's entry into what is considered the physician's private practice domain. The medical center also perceived a need to be able to deliver the "physician piece" in connection with hospital services as managed care opportunities present themselves and as the medical center attempts to contract directly with self-insured employers. In addition, the medical center has had difficulty recruiting physicians to fill gaps in its practice base, especially ob/gyn physicians and primary care physicians for rural satellites that it wishes to develop.

From these concerns and objectives, the medical center and key physicians have determined the need to develop a number of primary care center (PCC) satellites ringing the medical center in its primary and secondary service areas, all to be marketed and linked together with a common identification, and all to be capable of pursuing managed care opportunities along with more traditional aspects of primary private office practice.

Both physicians and the medical center have decided to approach this strategy on a joint venture basis in which physicians and the medical center will share in the planning, development, and operation of the venture, including its ownership, its governance, and its risks and rewards.

From the perspective of the medical center, it felt the need for physician participation in the venture (1) to ameliorate past criticisms by members of the medical staff; (2) to better manage a strategy that, in essence, will be based on the private office model; and (3) to secure the commitment of a wide universe of physicians. From the physician's standpoint, the medical center's participation was also essential, among other things, because of the significant capital that would be required to secure the referral-base objective of the PCC strategy.

The implementation of the PCC strategy involved the creation of two new entities: the ambulatory services organization (ASO) and the network medical group (NMG) (see figure 4.6). The ASO in this example is a general partnership owned jointly by the medical center and by the physicians through the NMG. The ASO was organized as a general partnership for tax and simplicity reasons, given the fact that it has only two owners, the medical center (or its affiliate) and the NMG. Because of the large capital required, the medical center is the majority owner of the ASO and is entitled to a commensurate, major share of its return on equity. However, the NMG has been given an option over five years to purchase a larger interest in the ASO on defined terms and conditions.

Figure 4.6. Sample Primary Care Strategy Involving a Joint Venture

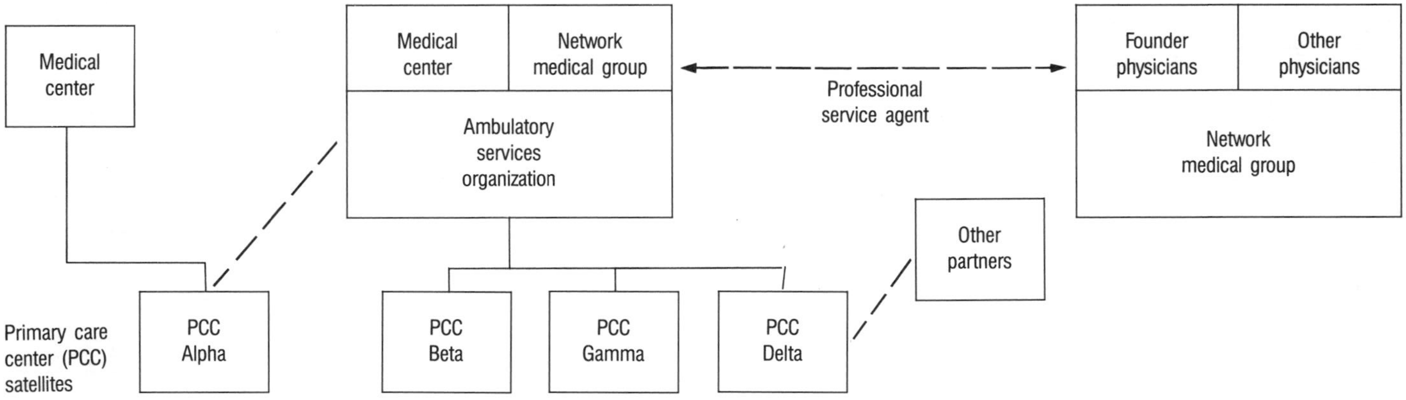

Moreover, the medical center has agreed to share governance in the ASO with the NMG in a manner disproportionate to relative ownership, with the objectives of securing strong physician participation and commitment. Specifically, a management committee was created consisting of three physician representatives of the NMG and only two medical center representatives. However, this governance representation is coupled with defined powers reserved for the medical center. In addition, specific ground rules have been established in joint venture guidelines dealing with such subjects as matters to be covered by the joint venture, opportunities that can be pursued by either party independent of the joint venture, and opportunities that must be offered first to the joint venture on a right-of-first-refusal basis.

This coupling of governance, reserve powers, and joint venture guidelines gave the medical center sufficient comfort to proceed with the joint venture PCC strategy even though it did not have a majority control of the management committee. In reaching this position, the medical center was strongly influenced by the desire to obtain the full commitment of participating physicians.

The medical center transferred its urgent care centers to the ASO for the appraised value, except for PCC Alpha, which it agreed to have the ASO operate on a management contract basis. A new satellite (PCC Delta) was established in a rural area on a joint venture basis; the ASO serves as a general partner in a new limited partnership, and local investors in the real estate serve as limited partners.

The ASO operates the satellites on a turnkey basis, providing all services except the physician services that are furnished by the NMG. The ASO's services include all facilities, equipment, personnel, and administrative support services. In addition, the ASO may contract directly with managed care programs and then subcontract with the NMG for physician services. The ASO may also furnish management and administrative services to unrelated physicians.

The NMG provides professional coverage for all satellites through employed physicians or independent contractors. It was organized as a professional corporation, with founder physicians as the initial shareholders. However, other physicians were added soon thereafter, including a large, multispecialty group practice in town, as well as primary care physicians, specialists, and participating staff physicians. The NMG staffs the satellites through a combination of physicians it employs, including those whose practices have been acquired and independent contracting physicians. Back-up coverage is arranged through subcontracts with shareholder-physician groups in such areas as obstetrics-gynecology and pediatrics. The NMG uses a new provider billing number for Medicare and other third-party billing.

The NMG appoints and furnishes a medical director for the PCC strategy and is responsible for establishing and monitoring clinical policies for the satellites. It carries these responsibilities out primarily by contracting with several clinical directors, such as in the areas of internal medicine and obstetrics-gynecology. As physicians, NMG's medical and clinical directors are able to relate to the staff physicians and to oversee the office-based practices. Moreover, because the physicians have an economic stake in the ASO, they are sensitive to the number of satellites, their respective sizes, their levels of staffing, and their capital requirements.

A spin-off service of the NMG is to arrange for off-hour and back-up coverage for shareholder-physician practices. In addition, the NMG and the ASO are exploring the joint venture development of diagnostic elements of the satellites such as imaging and laboratory services. Moreover, discussions are now under way as to the use of this joint venture model to house other ambulatory care programs to be transferred by the medical center. Discussions are also examining the use of the ASO as the vehicle by which the medical center and its physicians can launch other programs.

This example illustrates the use of the joint venture approach to developing a PCC strategy and should be compared to the way a similar strategy is pursued by a hospital on a "go it alone basis," as is illustrated by figure 4.5. Either way is an acceptable solution to a primary care strategy whose key objective is the creation of a successful economic interdependence between the hospital and a large universe of committed physicians. The means selected will likely turn on political reality measured against the hospital's desire for ownership and control.

Control versus Participation

As illustrated in the preceding sections, the issue of control often becomes a determinative factor in selecting the organizational structure for the acquisition of practices in particular and for physician-hospital bonding in general. Too often this issue is presented as a "take it or leave it" proposition with a not unexpected, polarized, negative response. In fact, control is a composite of a number of factors, each of which can be analyzed on its own terms and perhaps allocated among the participants in a way that is broadly acceptable. For example, in a typical joint venture, control can be dissected into the following factors:

- *Ownership.* How is initial capital to be contributed? Should one or more classes of equity holders have the option to purchase larger interests over the course of time even if they are not financially able to meet the hospital's share initially? Can ownership be structured in separate classes to ensure minimum participation by specific categories of physicians such as primary care physicians, subspecialists, hospital-based physicians, and large, multispecialty group practices? Regardless of the ownership structure, will return on investment be directly correlated with the amount of capital contributed by each investor, or will certain investors receive a disproportionate rate of return?

- *Governance.* Is the governing body of the venture representative of the pro rata ownership interest, or does it reflect a disproportionate representation? This is an area where the hospital as an owner of a larger share of the venture may nevertheless be comfortable with broader physician participation on the governing body so as to secure a wide commitment from key referring physicians.
- *Reserve powers.* Again, if one party (for example, the hospital) retains ultimate authority through defined reserve powers with regard to a finite list of key issues, it may be more willing to have a smaller number of seats on the governing body even though it has a larger equity share.

In addition, control or influence can be secured in ways other than through ownership and board seats. These ways include:

- Leases, loan documents, and contracts containing certain conditions, covenants, and restrictions (CC&Rs), the default of which gives the holder thereof certain enforcement rights.
- Transfer agreements such as where the hospital transfers an existing ambulatory surgery program to a joint venture entity in which the hospital has only a minority of board seats. As a part of the transfer agreement, the hospital can require the joint venture to adhere to designated affirmative covenants, for example, giving the right to the hospital to include the ambulatory surgery center as part of its bid response to HMO contracting opportunities on a discounted price basis.
- Joint venturing guidelines where, as a "Magna Carta," the parties can agree to the fundamental principles governing the transaction including such things as a covenant not to compete, the violation of which may give rise to specified remedies.

Control can thus be approached in a variety of ways and need not be viewed as an either-or proposition. As such, the hospital-physician transaction can be structured to allow for the sharing of ownership, authority, and responsibility and, at the same time, to meet the different objectives and concerns of the hospital and physician participants.

Conclusion

This chapter suggested a number of ways to structure a hospital-physician bonding transaction, ranging from practice enhancement to acquisition of physician practices to a comprehensive hospital-physician joint venture development of multiple practice settings. The primary features of these alternative structures were described in order to provide guidance to hospitals and physicians as they approach specific transaction opportunities. However, it must be emphasized that it is of primary importance to develop a clear picture of the facts, or circumstances, behind the transaction; that is, the potential participants along with the objectives and concerns of each must be identified before an appropriate structure can be tailored to fit.

Notes

1. Robinson-Patman Act, 15 USC § 13a et. seq.
2. Risk Retention Amendments of 1986, Public Law 99-563.
3. This list of structural arrangements for practice acquisition is not exhaustive. A number of other legal arrangements can be relevant to this discussion. For example, in one such arrangement, organized physicians may "own" or control hospitals. An example of this arrangement is the recent merger of Rochester Methodist Hospital and St. Mary's Hospital of Rochester in Rochester, Minnesota, into the tax-exempt Mayo Clinic, whereby the Mayo Clinic became the sole corporate member of both tax-exempt hospitals and, as such, became their parent. Many hospital-physician relationships often involve such a blending of legal control and the practical, political ability to influence decision making. This blending permeates hospital-physician interactions on all levels and is not limited to practice acquisition transactions.

Chapter 5

Legal Issues

Ross E. Stromberg

A hospital that is examining the various structures under which it can acquire and enhance the practice of a physician is subject to a number of legal rules. Many of these rules address the compensation arrangement between the hospital and the physician and impose restrictions upon the manner and purpose of such compensation. The justification for some restrictions may be the protection of the public from unscrupulous practices such as kickback or referral fees for services or the practice of medicine by nonlicensed practitioners. Other restrictions may be designed to prohibit a hospital from acting in a manner contrary to the protection and benefits it receives because of its status under law. For example, a tax-exempt hospital needs to be cautious about the protection of its tax-exempt status. Other rules apply to due diligence whereby a hospital reviews the proposed transaction to assure itself that it is getting what it is bargaining for and that it is minimizing the possibility of subsequent surprises. Consequently, a hospital desiring to pursue an arrangement with a physician, whether it be an acquisition of a practice or another form of physician-hospital bonding, should first seek advice about laws and regulations that may be applicable to the proposed arrangement.

Medicare and Medicaid Fraud and Abuse Prevention

A provider under Medicare and Medicaid programs is subject to certain restrictions designed to thwart potential fraud and abuse. For example, Section 1877(b) (antikickback provision) of the Social Security Act prohibits the knowing and willful solicitation or receipt of any remuneration (including any kickbacks, bribes, or rebates) or the offering or paying of any remuneration, directly or indirectly, overtly or covertly, in cash or in kind:

- In return for referring an individual to a person for the furnishing or arranging for the furnishing of any item or service for which payment may be made in whole or in part under Title XVIII, Social Security Act, or
- In return for purchasing, leasing, ordering, or arranging for, or recommending purchasing, leasing, or ordering any good facility, service, or items for which payment may be made in whole or in part under Title XVIII.[1]

The Medicaid program contains an identical prohibition.[2]

This restriction on fees is not applicable to all situations. For example, the law specifically exempts discounts or reductions in price obtained by providers if the reduction is properly disclosed and the cost is claimed or the charges made by the provider.

In addition, a key exception applicable to the acquisition of physician practices is the specific exemption for amounts paid under a bona fide employer-employee relationship.[3] There is legislative history that suggests that this exception is applicable to an agency or other comparable arrangement in addition to strict employer-employee relationships, although the scope of this exemption has never been tested.

In addition to the federal antifraud and abuse provisions, there may be comparable state-law restrictions that the hospital and its physicians should keep in mind. For example, California's Medical Practice Act broadly defines an unlawful referral fee as "any rebate, refund, commission, preference, patronage, dividend, discount, or other consideration, whether in the form of money or otherwise, as compensation or inducement for referring patients . . . to any person."[4]

A provider who engages in activities in violation of the Medicare and Medicaid prohibitions on referral fees may be punished with either fines of up to $25,000 or imprisonment of up to five years or both. Furthermore, a provider who is convicted of such a violation may be excluded from participation in the Medicare and Medicaid programs.[5] Finally, on enforcement, no payment may be made by the Medicare program for any item or service furnished by physicians or other individuals barred from participation in the Medicare program under these provisions.

Unfortunately, little practical guidance is available through case law or through the agencies responsible for the enforcement of the antifraud and abuse provisions with respect to physician practice acquisition strategies. The two primary enforcement agencies are the Office of the Inspector General of the Health Care Financing Administration (HCFA) and the U.S. Department of Justice. Because of the criminal nature of the federal antifraud and abuse legislation, neither agency has authority to issue advisory opinions.

While legislative history suggests a primary concern over blatant abuses such as Medicaid "mills" and kickbacks for laboratory referrals, the language of the legislation is so broad that it indeed can have a chilling effect on many arrangements between hospitals and physicians that otherwise may seem quite legitimate. Unfortunately, this chilling effect is accentuated by the decision in *United States v. Greber* (760 F.2d 68 [3rd Cir. 1985]), which demonstrates that despite the legislative history, the antifraud and abuse amendments could have potentially broad implications. The *Greber* case involved payments by a supplier of halter monitors to referring physicians allegedly as fees for interpretive readings performed by the referring physicians. The court holding was extremely broad in its conclusion that even though payments to a referring physician may be for professional services rendered, the payments nevertheless violate the antifraud and abuse amendments if "*one purpose* of the payments was to induce referrals." Most commentators, despite *Greber*, feel that if there is a legitimate business purpose for the transaction, it should stand the test of investigation even though an incidental effect of the relationship would be the enhancement of referrals. For that matter, all relationships between hospitals and physicians are designed to encourage cross referral of services, and to ignore this by literal application of the antifraud and abuse amendments seems to fly in the face of reality.

Suspect Arrangements

Nevertheless, many circumstances associated with physician practice acquisition strategies raise potential antifraud and abuse issues. These include:

- Requiring the physician who receives practice enhancement services to refer all patients to the hospital or its specialty staff, as a part of a written agreement.
- Requiring the physician whose practice is acquired to refer all patients to the hospital and its specialty physicians.
- Tying compensation or other forms of remuneration to the physician to the number of referrals actually made to the institution. Even if compensation is not specifically tied to the volume of referrals, a remuneration package may be suspect, such as when a medical director receives inordinately excessive compensation when compared to the service he or she renders.
- Tying return on investment by physicians in a joint venture, such as a practice management company, to the number of referrals made by the physician rather than to the amount of funds invested.
- Terminating compensation or other forms of remuneration because admissions or other referrals did not meet predetermined expectations.
- Tying forgiveness of loans to the number of referrals made to the institution.

The key factor in these circumstances is that a physician is mandated to make referrals to the institution in exchange for an economic consideration. Not all such arrangements are suspect. The test is to establish a bona fide, separate business justification for the arrangement and the payments made thereunder.

Possible Permissible Arrangements

There can be permissible arrangements under the antifraud and abuse amendments. These include:

- Tying compensation of physicians participating in acquired practices to services rendered by the physician or to the overall volume of the practice without regard to specific referrals to the hospital.
- Tying compensation of a medical director in a related group practice to the aggregate economic success of the practice. However, what if the medical director was also compensated on the basis of the volume increase of business to the sponsoring hospital? This at least raises questions in light of the literal application of the antifraud and abuse provisions.
- Requiring medical staff membership as a condition of participating in a joint venture. This is probably permissible, although to our knowledge it has not been tested. However, if the venture attempts to preclude membership in other medical staffs, this may be viewed as a prohibited indirect mandate of referrals.

New federal legislation, the Medicare Quality Protection Act of 1986 (PL99-509), prohibits physician incentive plans that reward a physician for reducing the length of stay or that target an amount of services rendered to a Medicare payment. The legislation also provides for additional civil penalties for the offending physician or hospital or for a Medicare Risk HMO/Competitive Medical Plan.

As indicated, the application of the antifraud and abuse amendments to the acquisition of physician practices is cloudy. There clearly are practices that would be prohibited, such as mandating referrals; but other practices are not so easily labeled as improper, such as tying compensation to the overall economic success of the venture. The antifraud and abuse issue should also be discussed in the context of what the entities hope to accomplish and how critical or integral the interdependence between the hospital and the physician is to the success of the venture. For example, hospital-based physicians are often required to limit their practice to that institution. The effect of this, of course, is to mandate exclusive use of hospital resources. Similarly, the very nature of a health maintenance organization (HMO) is to lock in providers and compel the use of panel physicians or panel hospitals with the consequence that benefits furnished by nonparticipating providers would not be compensated. This has never been challenged, to the author's knowledge, as a violation of antifraud and abuse amendments even though it mandates referrals. Presumably, this practice can be supported by acknowledging that mandating referrals in an HMO is an integral part of an HMO's operations. The question then is whether this kind of argument can be made to support a program of anticipated referrals in a physician practice enhancement or acquisition program. Again, if there are legitimate business purposes for the relationship, as opposed to a bold referral fee or kickback, the practice may withstand close scrutiny. The problem here is that there have been few, if any, cases directly applicable to hospital-physician bonding, and this fact, coupled with the inability of the enforcing agencies to give advance advisory opinions, gives us little in the way of guidance to lead the way through this thicket.

Corporate Practice Acts and Professional Licensure Requirements

The Corporate Practice Acts present some major legal issues for many hospitals as they explore the acquisition of physician practices.

Permissible Aspects of Practice Acquisition

One key issue is whether a hospital can purchase the clinical aspects of a physician practice, that is, patients, patients' records, and practice goodwill as distinguished from only hard assets such as real estate and equipment. For those states allowing a licensed hospital to employ a physician on a salary basis, there should be little difficulty from a legal standpoint under the medical practice acts as to the hospital's purchasing the clinical aspects of a practice and paying compensation therefor. After the acquisition, the physician could become an employee of the hospital, and, in essence, the hospital would be conducting the private practice of medicine.

However, states such as California, Ohio, and Texas prohibit the direct employment of physicians on a salary basis by hospitals, with notable exceptions to this rule. In each of those states, arguably licensed hospitals may not purchase the clinical aspects of a practice unless the transaction falls within one of those exceptions. Clearly, such hospitals cannot employ physicians and, therefore, cannot acquire patients, patients' records, and practice goodwill. Hospitals in such states may arguably purchase only the nonclinical aspects of the practice, such as real estate, equipment, and personnel, and must make other arrangements for the transition of the clinical aspects of the practice, such as to a friendly, multispecialty group practice.

Even in states where the employment of physicians is prohibited as the illegal corporate practice of medicine, the law has generally not been tested in modern times and basically reflects old cases and attorney general opinions growing out of the 1930s' concern for "department store medicine." Thus it remains to be seen how a hospital's acquiring a physician's practice today would be viewed by legal authorities in such states.

In states where licensed hospitals can employ physicians, a second question is whether it is permissible for an affiliated entity of a hospital to purchase the clinical aspects of the physician's practice. For example, suppose that the acquiring entity is not the hospital itself but rather the parent holding company of the hospital or a sister corporation to the hospital, neither of which is licensed as a hospital facility. Is the exception to the corporate practice rule limited to the licensed hospital itself, or would it apply to any affiliate of the hospital? Similarly, some states make a distinction between for-profit and not-for-profit health-related entities and only allow the latter to employ physicians.

Oftentimes the issue of corporate practice is stated in the context of whether a hospital or other entity can employ physicians on a salary basis. Perhaps a more logical way of stating this issue is whether unlicensed lay persons are improperly interfering with the physician's clinical decision-making authority. In the author's view, this is the only appropriate, underlying rationale for the prohibition against the corporate practice of medicine. It should matter little whether a physician is employed by a hospital, for-profit or not-for-profit, or by another physician or large group practice; rather, the question should be: Are any unlicensed persons improperly interfering with the physician's ability to exercise medical judgment? If that interference exists, the practice of medicine becomes corporate and illegal. If that interference does not exist, the question of whether the physician is an employee or independent contractor should be legally irrelevant.

Management Fees as Fee Splitting

Another key issue of corporate practice is whether the hospital's (or affiliate's) furnishing services, equipment, supplies, and personnel to a physician practice and receiving as compensation a percentage of gross or net income constitutes improper fee splitting under state medical practice acts. Generally speaking, a percentage of net income is more suspect than a percentage of gross arrangement. The overall test is the reasonableness of the compensation received for the services rendered, not the format of such compensation.

Management of Practice as Illegally Controlling the Practice

A related question is whether the interrelationship between the hospital or the affiliate and the dependence of the physician on services received is so pervasive that it amounts to an indirect control of that practice. See, for example, *California Association of Dispensing Opticians v. Pearle Vision Center* (143 Cal.App.3d [1983]), which held that in a dispensing optician franchising situation, the control by the franchiser company was so pervasive that it amounted to the corporate practice of professional services.

Other Practice Act Considerations

Other considerations under the medical practice acts include:

- Limitations on the use of names by medical practices or clinics, and registration requirements with state medical practice agencies.
- Limitations on a professional corporation's owning stock in other professional corporations. Generally speaking, only individual practitioners can be shareholders in professional corporations. This limitation should be taken into account as multiple acquisitions are made.
- The ability of a nonphysician entity, such as the hospital or an affiliate, to influence the transfer of stock of a related professional corporation from one shareholder to another, such as when the single shareholder of the related group practice, who was the medical director of the program, no longer serves in that position.
- Disclosure requirements, that is, state laws mandating disclosure of a physician's economic interest in any health care facility or service to which he or she refers a patient. In that regard, see also the various ethical pronouncements by the American Medical Association and other professional societies generally requiring disclosure on the part of practitioners of economic interests in referral arrangements. In addition, see the companion requirement that the physician must always be guided by what is best for the patient's medical interest.

Other Licensing Considerations

Related licensing considerations should also be taken into account. For example, does the acquisition of a medical practice require a certificate of need? This is probably unlikely in most states, but if the program is of sufficient magnitude or is viewed to involve the establishment of new services, a certificate of need may be required in certain jurisdictions.

Another licensing question is whether the acquired practice must be licensed as part of the hospital or as an outpatient department of the hospital, or whether it should be licensed as a freestanding clinic. Some states such as California provide a separate clinic licensing status, and that may have some advantages or disadvantages as an alternative to a practice's being treated as a hospital outpatient department or as a private office practice.

Tax Considerations

A transaction by a hospital to enhance or acquire a physician practice should be examined carefully for its tax implications both for the hospital and for the physician involved.

Private Inurement and Private Benefit Standards

If the hospital is tax exempt, any transaction in which it purchases a practice or pays consideration to a physician (for example, in the case of recruitment assistance or income guaranties) must be analyzed for potential jeopardy to the hospital's tax-exempt status. Tax-exempt hospitals and affiliates that are exempt under Section 501(c)(3) of the Internal Revenue Code (including a parent holding company) are subject to the requirement that they be "organized and operated exclusively for religious, charitable, [or] scientific . . . purposes, . . . no part of the net earnings of which inures to the benefit of any private shareholder or individual."

The phrase "net earnings" is broader than net income and is not limited to improper distribution of dividends. Rather, the prohibition against private inurement applies to any situation in which a tax-exempt entity transfers its cash, property, or other assets to an "insider" (for example, a person who has a personal and private interest in the charity) without adequate consideration. Tax-exempt status may be revoked upon any finding of private inurement without regard to amount.[6]

As a technical matter, the doctrine of private inurement is limited to payment of net earnings to so-called insiders and does not include payments to unrelated third parties.[7] Nevertheless, the Internal Revenue Service has taken the position that medical staff members are insiders for purposes of applying the prohibition against private inurement.[8]

Regardless of whether a physician is properly treated as an insider for purposes of applying the private inurement test, there is, in addition to the prohibition against private inurement, a requirement that tax-exempt hospitals be operated for the public benefit and not for the benefit of any private individuals.

While there may be differences between the private inurement and private benefit standards, they appear to be roughly equivalent in general purpose and function. In this regard, one important consideration under both doctrines is fair value: Did the hospital receive a *quid pro quo*? Nevertheless, under the private benefit test, the IRS has recognized that tax-exempt organizations, in serving the public welfare, must necessarily benefit private individuals at times. The general counsel of the IRS has opined that such private benefits are acceptable so long as they are only "incidental." An acceptable incidental private benefit must be incidental in both a qualitative sense (that is, the benefit to the public cannot be achieved without necessarily benefiting certain private individuals) and in a quantitative sense (that is, the benefits must not be substantial when measured in the context of the overall public benefit).[9]

Many arrangements associated with physician practice enhancement and acquisition strategies raise potential private inurement and private benefit issues. These include:

- Office space leases where facilities or equipment are provided at little or no cost or at below market rates. To support such an activity, the hospital must show a nexus between the special arrangement and the hospital's charitable purpose.
- Working capital or capital asset acquisition loans, or guarantees of such loans. Again, if loans are provided at no interest or at a rate below market rate, or at least below the rate at which the hospital secures its own capital, such transactions may jeopardize the tax-exempt status of the hospital. In addition, if a loan is made at below the applicable federal rate of interest, income may be imputed to the borrower.[10]
- Income guarantee programs. A nexus must be shown to exist behind such a program and a hospital's charitable purpose.
- Excessive compensation arrangements. Salaries, fringe benefits, and other payments for services rendered result in private inurement or private benefit if they exceed the value of such services. Again, the question is one of *quid pro quo* and whether the compensation is excessive in light of the services rendered to the charity. This may be an issue of certain medical directorships particularly if compensation paid by a hospital to the physician is not matched by services received from the physician. Another potential problem exists where compensation is based in part on the net income of the tax-exempt entity.

While it is easy to state the general rule, it is difficult to apply it in particular cases. In General Counsel Memo 39498 (January 28, 1986), the general counsel of the Internal Revenue Service opined that a hospital's tax-exempt status may be jeopardized by a physician recruitment program that includes a two-year minimum income guaranty. The general counsel's objections seemed to stem more from the factual posture of the case than from any objections in principle. In fact, the general counsel conceded generally that hospitals must offer incentives to attract qualified physicians and found that the two-year income guaranty did not "on its face" pose any obstacles. The general counsel concluded, however, that it had not been demonstrated, nor did it seem possible to demonstrate, that all possible subsidies under the program were reasonable in terms of the benefits a recruited physician may bring to the hospital and its service area.

This ruling is important because it points out the need for a hospital contemplating a physician practice enhancement or acquisition program to do its homework, including a full analysis of a proposed transaction's private inurement and private benefit implications. The hospital's conclusions and rationale should be carefully documented for the record, explaining how the transaction would benefit the hospital in furthering its charitable purpose. Moreover, each transaction should be carefully described in written documents to clearly spell out its provisions and the responsibilities of the hospital. The Internal Revenue Service is concerned about the "open-endedness" of some transactions. This concern points out the need to cap or fix the outer limits of any compensation or comparable package of physician enhancements. Finally, all such programs should be presented to the hospital's governing body for approval or should at least be within clear, overall guidelines that have been established by the governing board.

Generally speaking, most practice enhancement or acquisition strategies can avoid the restrictions against private inurement and private benefit if the hospitals and physicians are mindful of these rules as they negotiate and implement their transactions.

Unrelated Business Income

Engaging in unrelated business activities to "more than an insubstantial part" of a tax-exempt entity's total activities may endanger the entity's tax-exempt status.[11] Even if the tax-exempt status is not jeopardized, income from unrelated business activities is subject to taxation at ordinary corporate rates. The appropriate test is whether an activity of a tax-exempt entity is substantially related to its public or charitable function, aside from the charity's need for financial support. If not, the income from the activity will be taxed as unrelated business income. An activity will be deemed unrelated if it does not "contribute importantly" to the accomplishment of the organization's tax-exempt purpose.[12]

In the context of enhancement or acquisition of physician practices, the unrelated business rules will likely apply to the sale of management and administrative services by a tax-exempt entity to a physician. However, provision of such services will not be subject to unrelated business income taxation as long as a nexus can be shown between the services rendered and the furtherance of the tax-exempt entity's charitable purpose. For example, income from support services rendered to physicians occupying a hospital's medical office building may not be deemed unrelated business income if close proximity of the physicians to the hospital arguably enhances the ability of the hospital to carry out its charitable purpose. Again, the hospital must document the underlying rationale for each management and administrative service so as to avoid unanticipated taxation issues.

Some forms of income that would otherwise be treated as taxable unrelated business income may not be subject to tax if the income comes from an investment-type activity such as real property rentals, interest income, or dividends from a corporation in which the hospital is a shareholder. However, there are many exceptions to this rule, such as where the rent payer is controlled by the hospital or where the so-called debt-financed rules apply. These rules require that the hospital include as an item of unrelated business income any income from debt-financed property, which is property that is acquired or improved by means of incurring indebtedness. [13]

Allocation of Purchase Price in the Acquisition of a Physician's Practice

Traditionally, sellers wanted, for tax reasons, to maximize the allocation of the purchase price to assets that generated capital gain, whereas purchasers wanted to maximize allocation of the purchase price to assets that could be expensed or rapidly depreciated or amortized. Such objectives were generally in conflict, and the Internal Revenue Service, as a result, would often respect allocations made by buyers and sellers in such arm's-length negotiations.

Examples would be situations in which sellers, on the one hand, wanted to maximize the allocation of the purchase price to goodwill (all capital gain, but nonamortizable and nondepreciable) or to real property (generally capital gain, but extended depreciation only). Purchasers, on the other hand, wanted to maximize the allocation to inventory, which could be expensed, to equipment (ordinary income up to recapture amount, but rapidly depreciable), or to covenants not to compete (all ordinary income, amortizable over the term).

However, given the elimination by the Tax Reform Act of 1986 of different tax rates for capital gains and ordinary income, the objective of the parties may now be more consistent, with the seller agreeing to maximize allocation of the purchase price to inventory, to equipment, and to covenants not to compete. As a result, the Internal Revenue Service may not be as willing in the future to accept these allocations because the parties no longer have conflicting interests regarding the allocations.

Nevertheless, some of these allocation decisions may still be important, particularly where a selling physician has capital losses that he or she needs to offset capital gains in order to deduct such losses. In addition, sellers receiving consideration in cash or cashlike property may wish to avoid immediate recognition of gain or loss and thus may seek to negotiate the transaction on an installment-sale basis.

The purchase of practices by not-for-profit hospitals does not qualify for any tax-free exchanges (such as mergers or transactions in which the stock or assets of a physician practice are exchanged for stock in the acquiring corporation). Nevertheless, such opportunities would be available if the acquiring entity were a for-profit subsidiary of the hospital.

The Tax Reform Act of 1986 eliminated tax credits such as investment tax credits and extended depreciation periods for most types of property. Thus there may be little in the way of tax benefits through capital investment in the acquisition of practices. This points out what always should have been the case: the need to structure any such arrangement on economic rather than tax-benefit reasons.

Charitable Trust Doctrine

Laws of all states generally hold that assets of a charitable organization are impressed with a charitable trust and are not to be used in a manner contrary to the charitable purpose as expressed in the organization's basic charter or otherwise. Thus the use of a tax-exempt hospital's assets to confer a private benefit upon a physician could be deemed a breach of the charitable trust doctrine. The attorney general in each state is generally empowered with the ability to enforce the charitable trust doctrine and could bring an action to recover any asset impermissibly transferred to a physician by a tax-exempt hospital.

The preceding discussion concerning private inurement or private benefit standards under the Internal Revenue Code is generally applicable to the consideration of a potential violation of the Doctrine of Charitable Trust. Note, however, that these are two separate doctrines enforced by two separate agencies.

Employee Retirement Income Security Act Considerations

Two aspects of the Employee Retirement Income Security Act (ERISA) could be pertinent to the acquisition of physician practices. These are the Affiliated Service Group Rules under Section 414(m) of the Internal Revenue Code and the Leased Employee Rule under Section 414(n) of the Code.

Section 414(m) Affiliated Service Group Rules

Under ERISA, employee benefit plans such as pension and profit-sharing plans may qualify for or may retain tax-exempt qualified status only if they do not discriminate in favor of owner-employees or other highly compensated employees when compared to rank-and-file employees. Over the years, persons have attempted to avoid the so-called antidiscrimination rules of ERISA by conducting business through multiple business entities. Congress responded to this loophole with laws that require "affiliated employers" to be aggregated or treated as a single employer in defined circumstances for purposes of testing compliance with the antidiscrimination and various other ERISA qualification rules. Under the Affiliated Service Group (ASG) Rules, all employees or members of an ASG must be treated as having a single employer for ERISA purposes. An ASG is defined as:

- A service organization, typically referred to as a "first service organization" (FSO); and
- One or more of the following:
    (1) Another service organization (an "A-Organization") if:
        (i) It is a shareholder or partner in the FSO, and
        (ii) It regularly performs services for the FSO or is regularly associated with the FSO in performing services for third parties; and/or
    (2) Any other organization (a "B-Organization") if:
        (i) A significant part of its business is the performance of services for the FSO or an A-Organization, which services are historically performed by employees, and
        (ii) It is 10 percent or more owned by officers, highly compensated employees, or owners of the FSO or an A-Organization.[14]

An organization may be a corporation, partnership, sole proprietorship, or any other business entity regardless of form, except that a corporation (other than a professional corporation) cannot be treated as an FSO with respect to an A-Organization.[15]

The applicability of the ASG Rules, which are admittedly complex, to physician practice enhancement and acquisition strategies is not crystal clear, due in no small measure to the unclear enforcement of these rules by the Internal Revenue Service in hospital-physician joint ventures and other relationships. Nevertheless, the rules could apply to the situation in which physicians have an ownership interest in the ambulatory services organization (ASO), that is, the organization that provides management or administrative services for its physician practices. Each physician practice could be deemed an FSO, and the ambulatory services organization could be deemed a B-Organization. The implications of these rules are that all such physician practices, along with the B-Organization, would be lumped together and treated like a single employer or an ASG for purposes of applying the antidiscrimination rules under ERISA. In short, the effect would be that if the rules are literally applied, the most lucrative pension plan of any one of the practices receiving such services would be deemed not to be a qualified plan unless the benefits of such a plan were made available on a comparable basis to employees of all affiliated practices in accordance with the ERISA antidiscrimination rules. The ASG Rules are illustrated in figure 5.1.

Figure 5.1. Affiliated Service Group Rules

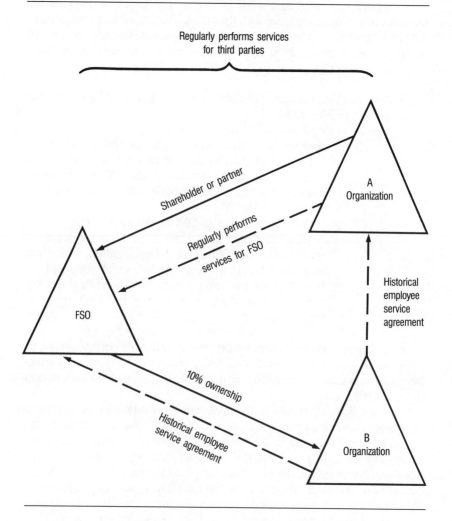

Note that there is a separate rule for management companies. An ASG may also consist of an organization whose principle business is the performance of management functions for one other organization (or related organizations) on a regular basis. [16] Thus regardless of the physicians' ownership of the ambulatory services organization, if the service bureau has been established to perform management services primarily for one physician practice entity, it and the physician entity may be deemed to be part of an ASG under ERISA.

Treatment of Leased Employees under ERISA

One likely service of an ambulatory services organization is the provision of personnel services to physician practices on a fee basis. Leased employees must be treated as employees of the lessee (the physician practice entity) rather than as employees of the lessor organization (the ambulatory services organization) for purposes of testing compliance with ERISA provisions where the services performed by the leased employees are the type historically performed by employees and where such services have been performed on a substantially full-time basis for at least one year.[17] There is a safe harbor to avoid the application of the Leased Employee Rule. Under this test, leased employees who would otherwise be treated as employees of the lessee would not be so treated provided the lessor organization makes available to such employees a money-purchased pension plan that has a nonintegrated employer contribution rate of at least 10 percent and that provides for immediate participation and for full and immediate vesting. However, the Tax Reform Act of 1986 makes the safe harbor exception unavailable as to any lessee whose leased employees make up more than 20 percent of the full-time employees. This, in effect, would preclude the safe harbor for most situations whereby physicians receive personnel services from a central manpower services bureau. The effect is that such employees would be treated as employees of the lessee if the lessee has a pension fund distinct from that of the ambulatory services organization.

Antitrust Considerations

Most physician practice enhancement or acquisition strategies would raise few antitrust considerations. For example, while price fixing can be a major issue in hospital-physician managed care joint ventures, it likely would not be raised often in situations where hospitals acquire practices. Presumably, if the hospital is operating private practices directly following acquisition and at the same time manages competing practices, the hospital could arguably be setting fees for its competitors under such management contracts, and thus the specter of price fixing may be raised. This, in itself, is somewhat farfetched.

Technically speaking, a Sherman Act Section 1 violation (illegal contracts, combinations or conspiracies in restraints of trade) or a Section 2 violation (monopolization, attempting to monopolize, conspiracy to monopolize) could be raised if an acquisition strategy were so pervasive as to improperly tie up or dominate specific markets.

Perhaps the most important antitrust consideration is the possible application of the Robinson-Patman Act to a hospital's furnishing or reselling supplies to physicians that it has purchased at a discount on the basis of its status as a not-for-profit, charitable organization.[18] The Robinson-Patman Act prohibits a seller of commodities from discriminating in price between different purchasers of goods where the effect may be to lessen competition substantially. There is a statutory exception for not-for-profit hospitals where the hospital purchases such commodities for "its own use." The question is whether a hospital's resale of such goods as part of the services furnished to physicians through its practice enhancement strategies is for its own use. Generally speaking, a not-for-profit hospital is prohibited from passing on such discounts to its physicians. However, price differentials based on legitimate market factors, as opposed to the not-for-profit discount exception, are permissible, such as a situation in which a hospital's group-purchasing arrangement receives volume-price discounts.

Any hospital engaging in a group-purchasing program for its physicians must not pass on or resell supplies purchased on the basis of the not-for-profit discount exception. In addition, the hospital should maintain records and inventories tracking and separating commodities purchased pursuant to the not-for-profit discount exception from those purchased on a volume-price basis without regard to the not-for-profit discount.

An issue related to antitrust that often comes up in the acquisition of a physician practice is the imposition of a covenant not to compete. Generally speaking, many states by statute or case law, in addition to the federal antitrust laws, impose limitations on proposed covenants not to compete in terms of their applicability to professional or personal services contracts. This is particularly so with regard to the length of time or geographical territory of the covenant. It is fair to say that the antitrust laws and many state courts view such restrictions on professional and personal services with a jaundiced eye. Before insisting on such a covenant, the hospital should carefully determine applicable state law as to the limits of such restrictions.

Medicare Reimbursement

Medicare reimbursement of hospital acquired or enhanced physician practices is often a key consideration in structuring the transaction. Questions concerning how physician services will be compensated under Medicare, and whether the practice will also be reimbursed for the hospital's technical component or "facility fee" must be considered.

General Rule of Physician Reimbursement

As a general rule, the services of physicians to Medicare patients are paid on the basis of reasonable charges under Part B of the Medicare program, unlike Part A, which pays hospital providers on a prospective pricing or reasonable cost basis. This payment methodology for physicians is subject to a 20 percent coinsurance requirement and deductibles.[19] If a physician is a salaried employee of a hospital or another provider, the physician's charge for identifiable services to individual Medicare patients must be based on his or her compensation arrangement for such services.

In addition, where the physician's services are performed, that is, in his or her office or in a hospital outpatient department, has an important bearing on Medicare's reimbursement of the physician's compensation. Medicare assumes that if the physician is performing his or her practice in a hospital outpatient department, the overhead costs (utilities, personnel, administrative services, and so forth) are borne by the hospital and covered by the hospital's reimbursement under Part A and should not be borne by the physician under Part B of Medicare. Thus physician reimbursement for a private office practice is reduced by 40 percent if the physician's services are performed in a hospital outpatient department. However, the hospital is eligible for a facility or technical component under Part A.

Facility Fee

Some acquired physician practice settings are eligible for a facility fee or technical component in addition to physician reimbursement. These include both inpatient and outpatient hospital-owned practice settings. Other qualifying situations include certified ambulatory surgery centers and hospital-affiliated ambulatory surgery centers. All other physician practice settings do not qualify for separate facility fee reimbursement; these include so-called freestanding outpatient centers such as urgent centers and emergency centers. They are treated as physicians' private offices, and all of their facility services are compensated only under the general rule discussed in the preceding section.

Reassignment of Part B Physician Payments

Another Medicare issue is whether a hospital or an affiliated entity may take assignment of Part B physician payments that would otherwise go either to the beneficiary or to the physician only. Generally speaking, the Medicare intermediary or carrier is prohibited from paying assigned benefits to other than the physician who provides the services. There are exceptions to this general prohibition, including a physician's employer, a health facility such as a hospital, and organized health care delivery systems such as medical group practices. These exceptions are important to keep in mind as arrangements are made to manage or acquire a physician's practice. A comparable issue should also be taken into account where a hospital and affiliate desires to serve as a billing agent for the physician. This is technically not a reassignment but, rather, payment in the name of the physician to the physician's billing agent where the agent's compensation is not related in any way to the dollar amounts billed or collected. In other words, a billing agent cannot be compensated on a percentage basis.

New Profile and Provider Number

A final reimbursement comment that is related to the acquisition of physician practices is the possible requirement of a new profile and provider number. For example, if a new practice entity is established, such as a professional corporation, to house the clinical aspects of acquired physician practices, this entity will likely have to establish a new Medicare provider number and be paid on the basis of a new and unique Medicare fee profile.

Liability and Insurance Issues

In assessing whether to acquire or enhance a physician's practice, the hospital should consider what the liability implications may be and whether such implications can be ameliorated through appropriate insurance arrangements.

Legal Responsibility of the Hospital for Physician Liability

Following the acquisition of a physician practice, a hospital or its affiliate may be held vicariously responsible for the allegedly negligent acts of the physician performing medical services even if the services are provided in nonhospital facilities. This will clearly be the case if the physician is an employee of the hospital or is deemed to be the agent of the hospital. Generally speaking, if the physician is not an employee but is, rather, an independent contractor, the hospital with whom he or she contracts will not be held vicariously responsible for the physician's alleged negligence.

Nevertheless, there are a number of exceptions to this independent contractor defense, such as where a court deems the relationship close enough to an employment relationship for purposes of applying the vicarious responsibility rules, or where the physician is viewed as an agent of the institution. Factors that are important in this consideration include: (1) the physician's lack of an independent private practice; (2) salary, vacations, or other fringe benefits that would suggest an employment relationship; (3) fixed hours of services; (4) the requirement that the physician adhere to rules and procedures of the hospital; and (5) the reasonable reliance of patients on the hospital as the overseer of the physicians assigned to such patients. The important lesson here is to be mindful of these trends and either distance the physician from the hospital or assume that there may be some responsibility for alleged negligent acts. You should take steps, through risk management programs, to minimize such occurrences, and you should insure the physician and the hospital adequately.

Insurance Considerations

Although the hospital's insurance covers the physicians, there may be a question as to whether the insurance is applicable to physicians who view themselves as independent contractors, notwithstanding what the courts may have to say about this issue. It may be prudent to seek endorsements to the hospital's policy in order to add physicians who are participating in the hospital's practice enhancement or acquisition programs.

As the malpractice insurance crisis continues to ebb and flow, a hospital arranging malpractice insurance for its physicians may be developing a very effective physician-bonding technique, which could be a determinative factor behind a successful physician practice enhancement or acquisition strategy. A brief discussion of this issue is in chapter 4.

Other Considerations of an Employment Relationship

The determination of whether a physician is an employee of or independent contractor to the hospital may be important for other considerations as well, including possible IRS requirements of withholding federal income taxes, social security, and state unemployment compensation. Similarly, this determination may be important for purposes of qualification under workers' compensation laws.

Due Diligence

An essential part of a physician practice enhancement or acquisition transaction is due diligence. From a buyer's perspective, due diligence means fully probing into the practice in terms of both operational and legal matters so that the buyer knows precisely what it is bargaining for and discovers problems that have to be addressed before the transaction is consummated. A buyer should also review its own status to ensure that the transaction does not violate any contracts or other obligations that preexist the transaction, such as its indenture.

In that regard, note that the Tax Reform Act of 1986 further limited the use of tax-exempt bond proceeds issued before the effective date of the Tax Reform Act for nonexempt activities such as medical office buildings or other assistance to physicians' private practices. Now under the Act, 95 percent of the net proceeds of a Section 501(c)(3) bond issue must be used in activities directly related to or essential to the conduct of the charitable activities of the hospital. This does not include funds used to finance an office building for use by physicians carrying on the private practice of medicine but could include the construction of hospital outpatient departments where physicians would not be conducting the private practice of medicine.

Another requirement of due diligence is to ensure that all requisite approvals of both the buyer and seller have or will be obtained before the transaction is consummated.

Conclusion

The legal concerns most likely to arise in a practice acquisition or enhancement transaction have been discussed in this chapter. It is important to note, however, that the unique circumstances of a transaction may give rise to other legal issues in addition to those discussed here. It is therefore critical to know the facts and circumstances of a proposed transaction. At that point, the participants and their legal counsel will be in a position to assess and resolve all of the pertinent legal issues in a timely and thorough fashion.

Notes

1. 42 USC §§ 1395mm(b)(1).
2. 42 USC §§ 1396h(b).
3. 42 USC §§ 1395(nn)(a)(3).
4. California Business and Professional Code § 650.
5. 42 USC § 1320 a-7(a) and (b).
6. *Spokane Motorcycle Club v. United States,* 222F. Supp. 151 (E.D. Wash. 1963).
7. Treas. Reg. §§ s 1.501(a)-(1)(c) and 1.501(c)(3)-(1)(c)(2).
8. See, e.g., GCM 39498 (January 28, 1986).
9. GCM 37789 (December 18, 1978).
10. IRC § 7872.
11. Treas. Reg. § 1.501(c)(3)-1(c)(1).
12. IRC § 513.
13. IRC § 514.
14. IRC § 414(m); Proposed Reg. § 1.414(m)-2.
15. Proposed Reg. § 1.414(m)-1(c)-2(e).
16. § 414(m)(5).
17. § 414(n).
18. *Robinson-Patman Act* (15 USC § 13).
19. See General CCH Medicare & Medicaid Guide, Paragraph 3185, et seq.

Chapter 6

Evaluating Candidate Practices

Steven Portnoy and Susan W. Wallner

Having developed the acquisition plan, reviewed the structural models and legal issues, and identified and met with a doctor who seems interested in the opportunity, you are ready to evaluate his or her practice.

Taking the Preliminary Steps

Let us begin by assuming that your initial meeting at this physician's office and the follow-up meeting at the hospital have caused you to feel that this practice offers real potential and that you will wish to acquire it if an in-depth evaluation shows it to be all you think it is. But before you can begin the evaluation, you need to exchange letters of intent in order to demonstrate the hospital's serious interest and to discourage the doctor from seeking other offers from competitor hospitals. You also need to show the hospital's good faith and encourage the doctor to display good faith as well.

Letters of Intent

You do not want to go through the time and expense of evaluating the practice until after the doctor has made a serious display of interest. Nor do you want to make an offer before the evaluation occurs. Incredible as it may seem, hospitals sometimes make dollar offers in order to interest the doctor in the concept before they really know what they are buying. When they later find out that their assumptions were wrong, they find themselves in a very awkward position.

Accordingly, a hospital's letter of intent should not include any anticipated components of the offer. Rather, the letter (usually signed by the CEO) should be a brief statement of the hospital's interest in the opportunity and its desire to develop an arrangement with the physician for the purchase of his or her practice, assuming a favorable outcome from the practice evaluation. Similarly, the physician should be requested to respond with a letter of intent signifying interest in the creation of an arrangement to sell his or her practice to the hospital. Such an exchange of letters of intent generally results in both parties' feeling that there is a preliminary meeting of the minds and a commitment to serious exploration of the details for a possible agreement.

Some hospitals require physician candidates to indicate in their letters of intent that they will not pursue the sale of their practice with any other hospital while the evaluation is taking place. Hospital advocates of "no-shopping" clauses say that unless they receive an up-front guarantee, they will not continue acquisition discussions with a physician. They feel that this is the only way to stop a physician from seeking other opportunities in order to play one hospital's offer against another's. Even if committed to writing, such no-shopping clauses sometimes work and sometimes do not.

Other hospitals do not believe in no-shopping clauses. They believe that, realistically, the physician agreeing to such a clause could still speak with other hospitals. In addition, a no-shopping clause could sour a physician toward the hospital because the clause could be viewed as an early indication that the hospital might be unreasonably controlling after purchasing the practice.

Displays of Good Faith

Following the completion of letters of intent, both parties would find it advantageous to show their good faith. The hospital could immediately offer temporary privileges to the physician if he was not already on the hospital staff. This would give the physician an opportunity to "try out" the hospital's services and determine whether he is likely to be happy practicing at the hospital. While being sensitive to legal and political boundaries, the hospital could also offer assistance to the physician with certain of his practice management or marketing needs. This would give him an example of how closely the hospital works with its medical staff, to their mutual benefit.

In return, the physician could begin admitting patients to the hospital or referring them to its specialists to show that he is seriously considering the opportunity. This would allow him to test the willingness of his patients to come to that hospital.

Such displays of good faith can sometimes lead to an early recognition by one or both parties that the marriage does not make sense. Having consulted on many physician affiliation arrangements, the authors have seen a number of potential marriages terminate quickly, despite good intentions, when the physician realized that his patients could not easily be persuaded to come to the hospital or that it was not convenient for the physician to do so either. Similarly, it is not unusual for a hospital to recognize quickly that a doctor does not fit in with its current medical staff or that the doctor will not be cost effective for the hospital under the diagnosis-related group (DRG) program.

Once the preliminary steps have been taken, your hospital should evaluate the practice thoroughly to assess the likelihood that it will fulfill the hospital's objectives on a long-term basis. The evaluation must review all aspects of the practice, ranging from strategic and operational aspects to financial worth. The following discussion highlights each of the major review categories.

Assessing Strategic and Operational Aspects of Practices

Most physicians want to keep the fact that they are considering selling their practice confidential until the deal is consummated. It is particularly important for the physician and the hospital to give some thought as to how the practice evaluator might be introduced to the physician's staff so that he can carry out his responsibilities. Perhaps the best choice is to introduce the evaluator to the office manager and staff as a practice management consultant who has been asked by the doctor to give him recommendations for the further development of his practice. The evaluator is then ready to begin assessing the strategic and operational aspects of the physician's practice.

Quality and Reputation

It is imperative that the evaluator assess the quality and reputation of the practice under consideration. The practice must not only meet the hospital's standards with respect to quality of care but must also engender a high level of patient satisfaction in order to contribute as a positive partner in the hospital's growth.

Physicians

The hospital should understand the number of physicians involved, their specialties and board certifications, and their other qualifications, as well as the more subjective qualities of personality, personal practice style, flexibility, and ability to develop a good rapport with patients. These qualities all contribute to the potential marketability of the practice.

In addition, the evaluator should help the hospital understand the current style of the practice as a whole. Such information as what the days and hours of operation are, which coverage arrangements exist, and whether the physicians maintain a hospital practice can influence the hospital's decision to acquire the practice, and can affect the specific terms of the acquisition contract.

It is also important to evaluate the long-range plans of the physicians who are either partners or associates in the practice. In a situation in which the principal physicians are planning retirement, the hospital must make sure that it understands the practice-time expectations of the physicians. It is advisable for each physician to continue his or her association with the practice, possibly on a less than full-time basis, for at least six months to a year following the acquisition in order to ensure a smooth transition, to introduce new physicians, and to maximize the probability that patients will remain with the practice.

Finally, the hospital should ascertain whether the goals of the principal physicians in the practice and hospital leadership provide a good fit. Two partners coming together with similar goals, practice philosophies, and long-range plans offer the highest probability of success.

Support Staff

Along with a consideration of the physicians within the practice, the hospital needs to evaluate the office's support staff. The number of full-time equivalents, their qualifications, and their ability to carry out their assigned tasks are also important assets to the practice. Similarly, the personalities, level of productivity, and ability of staff members to create and maintain a good rapport with patients enhance greatly the overall marketability of the practice. The evaluator should not fail to explore with support staff members, when the time is right, the likelihood that they will stay with the practice after its acquisition, both to ensure a smooth transition and to contribute to the stability of the practice.

The evaluator should obtain copies of job descriptions for the support staff to evaluate the appropriateness of tasks being completed in relation to the staff's qualifications. For example, some of the questions that the evaluator may wish to consider relate to whether certain tasks could be carried out by less-qualified ancillary staff members and whether the staff members are being utilized optimally. The evaluator should also explore employee benefits in order to help the hospital understand the expectations of support staff who may be asked to remain with the practice. Obligations to employees such as pensions, time off, and other requirements should be investigated.

Finances

For many organizations, the financial strength of a practice is the critical factor in the acquisition decision. From a careful study of tax returns, financial statements, journals, and other accounting worksheets, the evaluator can obtain a wide array of financial information that will address the following issues:

- Total revenue, with an understanding of whether this is expressed on a cash or accrual basis.
- Collection ratios, which give information not only on the credit worthiness of the practice patients but also on the billing systems and policies of the practice.
- Accounts receivable, which must be evaluated in light of the level of third-party coverage for the practice. Such information also reveals the credit profile of the patient base, as well as billing policies and financial health.
- Accounts payable, with attention to liabilities that may be assumed by the new owner of the practice, as well as to the cash control policies and procedures currently in place.
- Expenses, including an analysis of expenses that are personal.
- Payroll information, with information regarding overtime, bonuses, and pertinent practices and policies.
- Third-party reimbursement, with an examination of insurance statements that yield insurance profiles and fee schedule information.
- Overall profitability ratios, which may not only yield fiscal information but may also reveal strengths and weaknesses within the practice.
- Pension and other contractual obligations, with an understanding of those that will be acquired by the new owner.
- Other fiscal information, including all fee schedules, profit-sharing contracts, purchasing procedures, and so forth.

Patient Demographics

The hospital needs to know the demographic characteristics of the patient base currently being served by the practice. Understanding these demographics helps the hospital to evaluate the desirability of this market in relation to the institution's strategic business objectives and to determine whether the hospital can serve the clinical needs of the patients. For example, a hospital that does not offer obstetrical services may discover that a significant portion of a family practice patient base is composed of women of childbearing age.

To obtain information on patient demographics, the evaluator needs to study a significant number of patient records, reviewing perhaps 200 to 300 records over a period of the most recent two to three years. The number of records to be reviewed may vary per specialty. For an obstetrical practice, for example, a review of demographics for the previous five years is helpful.

Items of interest include residence locations of patients (with information regarding trends in the practice population over the time studied), the payer mix of the population (with similar attention to trends), and the socioeconomic mix of the patient base. This information includes the ages of patients, their educational and income levels (if available), the date of last visit, and other pertinent details such as employment data by types of occupation and employer. Information with respect to the date of last visit enables the hospital to evaluate further the activity trends within the practice. Employment information has particular significance for trends in insurance coverage within a community: Are major employers embracing managed care plans, which might affect utilization and revenue? Does the hospital participate in the plan(s) involved, and does such participation contribute to the hospital's goals, either fiscally or strategically?

To avoid buying the practice and finding out later that the doctor will come to your hospital but many of the patients will not, you need to understand the hospitalization preferences of the population currently being served. One mechanism to accomplish this is to conduct a brief research project, perhaps a questionnaire distributed to all patients seen in the practice for a 30-day period, which would query them as to the hospital of preference for a variety of services. You also need to know how patients travel to the office location, whether it be by private car, public transportation, or another mode. This can affect your hospital's decision to relocate the practice.

Attention also needs to be paid to the scope of diagnoses currently seen within the practice. Information regarding the clinical profile of the patients suggests the impact of the acquisition on the hospital with respect to both utilization and projected DRG income from this patient base.

Referral Patterns

The hospital should understand the historical referral patterns enjoyed by the practice. Both existing patterns and trends over time are significant in planning and decision making. Referral sources may include other physicians, other nonphysician health care professionals such as pharmacists, hospitals (through physician referral networks), emergency department or clinic rotations, other patients, and self-referrals.

Referral sources may also include prepaid provider organizations such as health maintenance organizations (HMOs) and preferred provider organizations (PPOs). The hospital must evaluate the practice's current level of participation, if any, in such plans, as well as the projected impact of any reasonably foreseen changes to existing contracts. The hospital also needs to understand the transferability of any contracts to the purchaser, as well as projected utilization and fiscal trends for the practice for each provider contract. For example, a hospital that has decided against participation in a particular HMO will probably find less value in acquiring a primary care practice in which some percentage of visits, and perhaps of revenue, results from participation in that HMO.

The hospital must consider not only historical trends in referral patterns but also the projected impact of acquisition upon them. For example, a specialty practice receiving a significant volume of referrals from primary care physicians affiliated with a competitor hospital may well see those referrals end upon acquisition. Nevertheless, the acquiring hospital may be confident in its ability to support the practice through its own referral channels. Whatever the conclusion, these issues must be thoroughly understood, as should issues relating to the impact of acquisition on physicians to whom the acquired practice has historically referred.

Market Analysis

The hospital must identify other providers within the marketplace, both competitors and friends. This knowledge is vital to the hospital's decision-making process. In a competitor-laden environment, the hospital needs to address whether it wishes to compete in a particular area. What degree of awareness of and preference for this hospital is evident in the market? Has this been evaluated by appropriate research techniques? Is the hospital willing to make an investment in influencing preference, if necessary?

The hospital may discover that its allies, either present members of the medical staff or other providers affiliated with "friendly" institutions, are active in the marketplace under consideration. Should that be the case, the hospital may be faced with a difficult decision. Will the hospital compete with its own medical staff in the community? Will it compete with other doctors on staff at other friendly hospitals? Even though the acquisition is not competitive in fact, will it appear to be competitive? What process has the organization selected to work through these issues? In some cases, a hospital may refrain from pursuing an acquisition opportunity rather than alienate a friendly physician or hospital.

Site Analysis

The hospital should understand the location of the practice and the availability of public transportation or main roadways to the site. Within the practice itself, the hospital needs to evaluate the amount of space available, the adequacy of space utilization, and the traffic flow within that space. The hospital should obtain a complete schedule of all furniture, fixtures, and equipment to remain with the practice, including inventoried supplies. The site evaluation should reflect not only the hospital's view of the practice but also a potential patient's view. Marketability includes such factors as visibility of the practice from the road, signage and restrictions (if any), as well as overall attractiveness, with attention to comfort and privacy within the office itself. If the building is owned by the physician, the hospital evaluator should ask for a complete tour in order to determine if there is value in purchasing the building.

Practice Operations

The hospital should understand the aspects of the practice's business operation that may affect the practice's desirability, value, and ability to fit with the hospital's own business procedures. This information includes functions of the reception desk (how the telephone is handled, how scheduling is accomplished), billing and collection procedures, inventory control measures, purchasing practices, and so forth. The hospital should obtain a complete set of relevant reports currently being generated by the practice – including accounts payable and receivable, aging schedules, and schedules of expenses – and information relating to personnel policies and procedures, including both payroll and benefits information.

Finally, it is critical that the hospital obtain information about all contracts, claims, and obligations of the practice. This includes information regarding lawsuits pending (both professional liability and others), liens, leases, pensions, and so forth.

Assessing Practice Value

Once the hospital has assessed the practice from the strategic and operational points of view, attention must turn to considering the value of the practice in economic terms. It should be remembered that the physician/seller will usually seek the highest possible value, and the hospital/buyer will seek the lowest value. The ultimate price to be paid lies somewhere in between. Techniques for selecting the price to offer will be discussed in the next chapter.

Many of the factors that are included in valuing the medical practice were also part of the initial decision to consider purchasing the practice. However, in this valuation phase, we will consider those factors from a purely financial standpoint.

The earnings of the practice over the past three years, together with an analysis of all sources of income, are of course given consideration in the valuation process. Gross income and net earnings are certainly important indicators of the success and growth of a practice. However, they do not provide any guarantee as to the productivity and profitability of the practice once it is purchased. For example, factors such as whether the physician stays with the practice, whether there are new competitive entrants into the practice marketplace, or whether the service area demographics change can influence the earnings potential of the practice.

Nevertheless, the hospital would be prudent to understand the earnings history of the practice, as well as which practice services generate those earnings. For example, in considering the purchase of a general practice, a hospital that maintains a discrete physical therapy service in the same geographic area may be surprised to find that a significant portion of the general practice's income is ascribed to physical therapy as well. At this point, the hospital must decide whether this service will continue to be included. However, if the hospital considers purchasing a practice that is not currently offering a particular type of testing, the practice may benefit from the inclusion of this product once the sale is consummated. If the hospital wishes to purchase the accounts receivable, the value of those that are collectible needs to be considered.

Similarly, the prospective purchaser needs to understand all of the expense areas of the practice. These include all overhead items such as salaries, rent, supplies, equipment, benefits, and so forth.

When evaluating sources of income, attention should be given to identifying referrers and referral agreements and contracts, if any, together with dates of expiration and transferability provisions. This enables the purchaser to develop educated projections regarding which activities will be retained after the acquisition, and it provides additional information regarding the overall financial impact of the purchase on the financial performance of the practice.

More specifically, decisions regarding participation in prepaid provider arrangements made either by the purchaser of the practice or by the managed care organization have a tremendous impact on the practice. A practice that has been heavily dependent in the past on such relationships for utilization and revenue will be of diminished value to a hospital that does not, or is not allowed to, participate in the same provider network.

Furniture and equipment need to be valued both from an economic and a practice-planning perspective. In itemizing each unit, professional valuators should consider the age and prospective life of the item, probable maintenance needs, and so forth. Clearly, the value of those items depends not only on their intrinsic worth but also on whether the purchaser wishes to put them to use in the practice.

The hospital should also find out whether any of the equipment within the practice is currently leased. Although leases are not ordinarily felt to be of value since leased equipment belongs not to the seller of the practice but to the lessor, a favorable lease that can be assumed by the buyer may be worth acquiring.

It is important to inventory both the medical and office supplies to be retained with the practice, as well as any quantity of medications that may be assumed by the buyer. Here buyer and seller should agree on a market value for these items, unless one overall price for the practice is developed.

The hospital should also consider whether there have been any leasehold improvements to the office, if the office itself is being assumed by the buyer. In some cases, leasehold improvements are indeed an asset. But in other cases, such improvements will revert to the landlord and, consequently, can be an expense item to the new owner if the landlord requires removal or restoration to the original state of the office. Similarly, the lease for the office space itself may be considered an asset if it is particularly favorable and is assumable by the purchaser.

Sometimes there is real estate involved with the practice, such as a condominium office suite or an owned building. If so, this needs to be dealt with as a separate real estate transaction, assuming the hospital is also interested in buying the property.

Other factors may affect the value of the physician practice. These factors, as covered earlier, include the practice's market share, new competition to the area, changing community demographics, and payer mix.

When evaluating specialty practices, two additional factors should be examined. First, the prospective purchaser needs to evaluate existing referral patterns and project the value of possible changes occurring as a result of the acquisition. For example, a neurology practice receiving 80 percent of its referrals for the past three years from six physicians on staff at Hospital B may experience the loss of those referrals upon acquisition by Hospital A. Second, attention should be paid to current and anticipated regulatory and reimbursement trends for that particular specialty in order to most accurately develop best-case and worst-case scenarios.

You have now completed the quantitative and qualitative evaluation of the practice being considered as a candidate for acquisition. If the results of the evaluation are favorable, it is time to develop the components and structure of the offer you will make to the physician.

Chapter 7

Creating and Negotiating the Offer

Steven Portnoy

The previous chapter reviewed the many factors you need to evaluate in a medical practice in order to determine if it is desirable for acquisition by the hospital and to enable you to assess the value of the practice. The present chapter explores options for pricing the practice and considers the other possible components of acquisition offers, which later become the terms of the purchase and sale agreements and the employment contracts.

The Components of the Offer

Determining the appropriate package to offer and negotiating the arrangement to successful closure both require thoughtful advance planning. Knowing the right amount to offer (both "going in" and as a "fallback") is essential for maintaining physician interest in the opportunity and for protecting the hospital's position.

Setting a Dollar Value

There is no one way to set a dollar value. As nice as it would be to have a simple formula for easily determining how much a practice is worth, such a solution does not exist, at least in this author's opinion. Despite the existence of formulas and rules of thumb, you also need to consider other factors when pricing a doctor's practice, which go well beyond numerics.

Areas for consideration in setting dollar value are:

- *The science of value setting.* This includes formulas and rules of thumb ranging from pricing each evaluated component of the practice and then totalling them to develop one overall price based on simple numerics. Some people value a practice at the most recent year's gross cash receipts or, perhaps, the average of the last three years' gross receipts. Others say that the starting point for negotiations is 50 percent of the annual gross cash receipts. Yet others look at 10 years' net profits. Some prefer offering a set amount of money per active patient record (considered unethical by some). And on, and on, and on. There are a variety of formulas used across the country, but none of these is more than a starting point.

- *The art of value setting.* Establishing a practice value that is both supportable and salable is more than a science; it is also an art. In addition to formulas, practice valuations often involve reason, emotion, and plain old guesswork. The dollar value of a practice is affected by considerations that have nothing to do with mathematics. "We will lose him to our competitor if we don't pay a bit more, maybe another $20,000." Or "despite what he says, this doctor is not likely to remain with the practice, and we should offer $15,000 less." Or "we have been having trouble finding out for sure, but I think this doctor has had some utilization problems at his current hospital; and if he comes here, we may lose money from some of his patients, so let's lowball him and offer 30 percent less than we originally had in mind."

- *The politics of value setting.* In addition to determining a value based on science and art, you must give recognition to political considerations. For example, the use of your preferred formula may indicate the value to be $165,000 for a particular practice. Applying art to setting value might dictate that this practice should only be priced at $135,000 because it appears that the doctor may really be more interested in semiretirement and slowing his productivity than in being active during the 18-month transition period you will require. But when you add in political considerations, that practice becomes priced at $115,000 or $175,000 or some other number because "we'd better pay the doctor less than we did Dr. A, but more than Dr. B. On the one hand, our loyal doctors would be unhappy if we gave him as much as Dr. A, who is an active physician and is well liked. On the other hand, we may lose the deal if the candidate finds out that we are paying him less than we did Dr. B."

Regardless of the intent to maintain total confidentiality expressed by both parties to the deal, you must always anticipate the word's getting out. Medical staff politics have often turned a practice acquisition upside down. Hence you should consider the political aspects of the dollar value set on a practice along with rule-of-thumb formulas, reason, and emotion.

Out of all of these considerations, the hospital comes up with a number that feels right. Before making the offer, though, the hospital should consider a fallback position. The hospital should set an upper limit beyond which it prefers not to go and should have this number in mind before meeting with the doctor to make the going-in offer. Candidates can sense pretty quickly how much room there is for negotiation. If a hospital appears to know what it is doing, the physician negotiators may not push too hard for fear of losing the deal and may be more flexible in their expectations.

In addition, the hospital should consider whether the dollar value that seems fair for the practice should or should not be the going-in amount to be offered. This question of negotiating strategy is often answered on the basis of the personalities of the CEO and other negotiators for the hospital and on their views of the physician's personality and likely strategy. You must try to read the thoughts of the other party before the negotiations begin. Some hospital administrators feel that some lesser amount should automatically be offered before negotiating up to what they really believe was fair in the first place. This strategy is often pursued where a CEO feels that a particular doctor will require an increase in the amount no matter what figure is quoted. Hospitals that believe a physician will milk an opportunity for everything it is worth often go to the other extreme and come in with an unrealistically low offer.

Yet other administrators believe, depending on their perception of a particular physician, that the wisest move is to immediately go in with a price that the hospital sees as the fair practice value. To do otherwise and offer an unrealistically low figure might result in the physician's becoming disenchanted with the hospital, leading him to consider another hospital's offer more seriously.

Considering the Concept behind the Acquisition

The dollar amount is only one component of the package to be offered. The terms of the offer and the nature of the arrangement should reflect the concept for the acquisition or, in other words, the "idea" that is behind the marriage. Is this a retiring doctor who will be replaced? Is the hospital acquiring the practice of a young doctor in a growing community in order to add partners, build a multispecialty practice, and market the satellite aggressively? The answers to questions such as these will drive the components of the offer.

For example, in addition to purchase price, language should be included in the contract requiring a retiring doctor to stay on for a period of time to help in the transition of the practice and patients to a new doctor. For a young doctor whose practice is being acquired, the arrangement should incorporate productivity incentives to ensure that adding new partners will not result in the physician's reducing his or her level of activity.

Thus the specific concept the hospital has in mind for each practice must be supported by the terms of the offer and the structure of the arrangement. Is the hospital interested in buying the practice in total or only certain components of the practice? On the one hand, if the reason for seriously considering a particular practice is to develop its potential as a major multispecialty and ancillary services satellite, the hospital is probably interested in buying the total practice. On the other hand, if the concept is simply to attract another doctor to the staff or to keep a current physician involved, the hospital may want to purchase only what it needs in order to satisfy the physician's interests. For example, the hospital may decide only to acquire the laboratory or radiology component of the practice.

If the hospital wants to use the practice location as a foundation for something bigger, the hospital may wish to buy the real estate. However, if the concept is to maintain the status quo with a physician already on staff in order to retain market share, the hospital may only want a lesser commitment, such as leasing the facility as a satellite clinic and contracting with the physician to provide medical services.

Determining the Logistics of the Transaction

Other components of the offer include the time period and nature of the payout, the employment and benefits package, and incentives. The hospital may wish to pay a one-time lump sum or may need to do so in order to meet a physician's expectations. The hospital may decide that it may be wiser, however, to pay out the purchase over three to five years, both to keep the physician involved and active and to spread out the financial impact for the hospital. If the latter course is chosen, the hospital may have to place a higher dollar value on the practice and finance it through the use of an annuity in order to still be able to sell the concept to the physician.

Another decision that needs to be made is whether the physician should become an employee with a base salary and perhaps a bonus or whether a contract should be provided for clinical services. The answer will depend on the physician's expectations and the hospital's motivations.

The hospital also needs to consider the benefits package to be made available to the physician. Insurance coverage, pension plans, vacation and holidays, opportunities to attend educational conferences, an automobile, and so forth, are all examples of what most physicians consider benefits they have always taken out of the practice, and which they will expect to be continued. Consideration should be given to whether incentives will be provided as part of the offer for maintaining quality and/or productivity. Since hospitals acquiring practices want to be sure that quality and productivity will not drop after acquisition contracts are signed, these hospitals may find it useful to provide incentives as part of the deal. This can take the form of a straight bonus, a percentage of net profits, a percentage of cost savings, and so forth.

Some hospital CEOs have great fun devising the components of an offer. It provides them with an opportunity to apply creative strategies to acquiring a valued asset through developing an offer that is most favorable to the hospital and that, at the same time, is satisfactory to the physician. For acquisitions to come to closure, a great deal of innovation is sometimes required on the part of the hospital team. If, for example, the CEO can sense that future security for the physician and his or her family is more important than the immediate availability of cash, the hospital may be able to obtain the practice at a lower cost by providing an especially attractive insurance or pension program for the doctor.

While some change in the physician's income, benefit structure, or practice style may be necessary to make the concept work, the fewer the changes the acquiring hospital requires of the physician, the easier it will be for him to agree to your offer instead of to one from a competing hospital. This author has on several occasions seen a higher dollar offer from one hospital fail to attract a physician who preferred a more creative offer from another hospital that was lower in dollar value, but required fewer changes to the practice.

Discussing Mutual Expectations

Some hospitals choose to limit their negotiations with the physician to the financial and structural aspects of the offer. They do not wish to discuss mutual expectations for, or changes in, the ongoing operation of the practice until after the deal is signed.

The reader is advised to take the other route and fully discuss the mutual expectations of the arrangement in advance of the deal's being signed. This will increase the likelihood of a long and happy marriage. Hospitals should speak openly with doctors and avoid pursuing acquisition opportunities that they think are likely to fail. If a hospital delays talking about expectations until after it signs the contracts, the physician may walk away after six months.

Questions recommended for discussion before signing contracts include:

- *What will be expected of the physician in terms of maintaining productivity within the practice?* How many hours a week will he or she need to be available? Will the physician be required to spend a certain number of hours teaching or otherwise working at the hospital?
- *How much freedom does the physician have to go outside the "hospital family"?* Assuming compliance with legal guidelines, will there be limitations on the physician's ability to admit or refer patients to other hospitals? Some acquiring hospitals expect all admissions and

referrals that they can care for appropriately to come to them. Other hospitals feel that their acquisition objectives will be satisfied if they are the recipients of the majority of a physician's patients. Rather than telling a physician that he will no longer be able to refer any patients to a specialist at another hospital who is his best friend and who he feels is competent in a particular field, the acquiring hospital may allow the physician to continue that long-standing relationship. The hospital does not want to chance having him walk away from the deal either before or after the contract is signed.

Most hospitals recognize that it would be unrealistic for certain patients from an acquired practice to come to them for hospitalization. Having evaluated the practice before making an offer, these hospitals can see that a percentage of the doctor's patients live too far from their facility, that some patients would not want to come to the particular area in which their hospital is located, or that for some other reason these patients might leave the doctor in favor of another physician if they were pressured to come to the acquiring hospital. These hospitals do not require 100 percent of the physician's patients to come to them.

In addition, most hospital attorneys advise their clients not to insist that all of a physician's patients be sent to them. Requiring a set number of admissions or referrals, restricting the free choice of patients to select their hospital, and demanding the admission of patients to a facility with limited subspecialties or a reputation for poor quality in a particular service are frequently cautioned against because they are legally questionable.

- *Who manages the practice clinically and administratively?* Some hospitals feel that a discussion of this issue in advance of signing the contract is inadvisable lest the physician be unhappy with what he or she hears. Others recognize that if the doctor is to be no longer in charge of the practice and is to come under a satellite medical director, he or she will probably prefer to discuss this up front rather than find out later and walk away after the deal is signed.
- *Will the hospital allow the doctor maximum independence, or will it oversee his or her activities closely?* Some acquiring hospitals view an acquired practice as an asset to be managed like any other part of the hospital. They intend to watch closely over the daily activities of the practice and to be involved with every decision. Other hospitals feel that pursuing this approach will hinder the long-term viability and success of the arrangement, for a physician who has been an independent entrepreneur making his own decisions for 20 or more years is not likely to appreciate being closely controlled all of a sudden.

Whichever approach is taken, you should discuss this issue in advance, especially if it will offer a competitive advantage for your hospital, which is seeking to outdo another hospital pursuing the same practice. If you intend to allow the physician to operate pretty much as he always has, and thus minimize his fears that the practice sale will mean he is no longer in charge, this should be made known to the doctor before he decides between an offer from your hospital and one from your competition.

- *What happens to the doctor's staff?* Some doctors do not care; others care very much. If you intend to change the doctor's staff, you should consider telling the physician before the deal is signed. Otherwise, there is the risk of quickly disenchanting a physician who suddenly finds out after signing the purchase and sale agreement that the office manager who has been with him for 19 years is to be let go. This can lead to a rapid deterioration in the relationship between the doctor and the hospital. If you discuss this up front and the physician objects, you can identify and work out options before the deal is signed, or you may choose not to pursue the opportunity further if you cannot come to an agreement.

- *Which office procedures will change?* Some discussion of this issue should be considered before completing the agreement. Certainly, not all details of all planned changes should be dealt with before signing the deal, for you do not want to complicate things unnecessarily. Some needed changes will not even be known to your hospital at that point. If a major change is to be made, however, you should discuss it with the doctor before completing the contract.

As you can see, while some acquisitions are very simple and straightforward, others require a great deal of time, effort, and money. The components of an arrangement can be complicated and can require much planning and negotiating. Although some hospitals may choose not to discuss mutual expectations, some will choose to do so, and others will be forced to do so by the physician. At the very least, the hospital team should consider discussing these expectations with the physicians before signing the contract.

Negotiating the Offer

Now that the hospital has decided on the components of the arrangement and has developed its offer, it can proceed with the negotiations. For most hospitals, though not all, the CEO is the lead negotiator. As was indicated in an earlier chapter, this primary negotiator needs to have the authority to alter the terms of the arrangement within a framework generally acceptable to the hospital's board. This individual should be present at all negotiating sessions so that the physician experiences consistency throughout the process. If a CEO feels that he or she needs help with the negotiations, consideration should be given to identifying another member of the acquisition team who can be actively involved or take the lead.

With regard to who negotiates for the doctor, it is common for many physicians to go beyond their attorneys for negotiation advice and support. Frequently, doctors also call upon their accountants, their consultants, their spouses, and their friends, in addition to their physician associates in the practice.

Regarding negotiations with a group practice, this author has gone through many a frustrating negotiation process with a three-physician or four-physician group in which each doctor is involved in the negotiations but the doctors alternate attendance at negotiating sessions with the hospital. Who attends the sessions is usually not planned but is more a function of who is available on a particular day or evening to meet with the hospital negotiating team. This can result in a tremendous waste of time and effort. It often leads to conflicting or confusing signals given by the physicians to the hospital, creating uncertainty as to how the hospital can satisfy their needs. If possible, the hospital should require that there be a lead negotiator for the physicians who can act as the spokesperson for the group.

Hospitals should involve their attorneys in reviewing the proposed offer before the negotiation process begins. While it is true that attorneys can complicate things, involving them in a carefully defined role in the negotiation process can help avoid confusion, misunderstandings, and violations of the law down the road. If the hospital has retained a management consultant to assist in the implementation of its acquisition program, the consultant should be available to offer support in the negotiating process as well. Like the attorneys, consultants should play a limited, advisory role in most cases. They can, however, be of great value in helping to overcome obstacles that may develop, based on their experience with other institutions acquiring physicians' practices. Consultants can also play a role with the physician after a negotiating session to help him or her consider the advantages and disadvantages of the opportunity. Decisions should be made on a case-by-case basis as to whether attorneys and/or consultants should attend the negotiating meetings with physicians.

When you reach what you thought was to be the final negotiating session, do not be surprised if you find out that the physician is still considering offers from competitor hospitals or brings up last-minute changes in the terms of the arrangement. Many doctors feel that it is in their best interest to seek other offers. This is especially the case with doctors who have not been on your staff in the past. Even physicians who have been active on your staff for many years and who have not considered other offers may have saved something until the last minute of negotiations. For example, some physicians will mention at the final session that "the books don't show everything." A certain amount of cash may have been pocketed over the years, which has somehow slipped through the practice accounting process. Or a benefit may have been provided by the practice that has not shown up on the books or the practice's records. A physician's spouse may have been traveling with the doctor to educational conferences in the Caribbean at the cost of the practice. A physician's children may have been working in the practice during school vacations answering the telephone. It is common for doctors to "remember" these past benefits at the last minute and to seek a dollar value for them as part of the final sale price or to request a guarantee that the activity can be continued.

If problems arise in the final negotiations, or if the negotiations turn out to drag on for six to nine months or even a year, do not automatically drop the opportunity. While this is frustrating and annoying, remember what the practice will be worth in terms of accomplishing the strategic objectives of the hospital. If the practice is not worth what you are experiencing, forget the deal. But if you still decide that it has great value, be patient. While some hospital executives and management consultants believe that any negotiations lasting more than 90 days should be terminated and the opportunity bypassed, this author has seen many very favorable outcomes from arrangements created after 9 to 12 months of negotiations. An artificial time limit should not be imposed on the negotiation period.

Remember that the physician is considering giving up his independence and selling a professional practice that he has developed over many years and of which he is very proud. Accepting this is not easy for the physician. Doctors appreciate hospitals that recognize and are sensitive to this fact and that are human as well as businesslike in their negotiations. Although the hospital is in fact purchasing equipment, supplies, patient records, and possibly real estate, it is not purchasing the physician or his patients. The physician must be happy about the opportunity in order to continue the success he or she has developed with a high level of energy and commitment to quality and productivity.

Chapter 8

Agreements

Ross E. Stromberg

Various ways of acquiring or enhancing a physician's practice were discussed in chapter 4. Each of these methodologies involves contracts between the parties, with attendant duties and obligations imposed on the parties by such agreements. Although each transaction must be crafted to fit the specific circumstances, the following discussion describes pertinent issues of the key documents that will likely be encountered in such transactions.

Agreements for Arrangements Short of Practice Acquisition

Administrative and Clinical Support Services

As discussed in chapter 4, strategies short of practice acquisition include the provision of administrative and clinical support services by the hospital to the physician. The objective is to enhance physician-hospital bonding without having to transfer ownership of the practice.

One vehicle to accomplish these strategies is to create a contractual relationship between the hospital and physician whereby specific administrative and/or clinical services are provided by the hospital to the physician. In addition to standard provisions, the agreement should clearly specify the scope and nature of services to be provided by the hospital. The discussions in chapter 4 highlight some of the management, administrative, and clinical support services that might be offered to physicians either as a complete managed practice or on a menued basis. The agreement should also define the timing of the services, that is, whether the services will be available on a daily, weekly, or monthly basis, and whether they will be provided on a project-by-project or ongoing basis.

Another important provision of the agreement involves a definition of who retains ownership of the products or services provided by the hospital. For example, if the hospital has the responsibility for furnishing computer hardware and software to link the physician to hospital terminals in order to track patients and ease the medical record keeping of the physician, would the physician or the hospital retain ownership of the software created to accomplish this goal? What if the hospital were responsible for providing billing and collection services to the physician and created specific software to perform those services? The key objective for the hospital would be to retain ownership interest in the software packages so that the hospital would be in a position to use the software for other physician practices. This raises another issue that should be addressed in the agreement: How exclusive should it be? Obviously, the hospital does not want to be prohibited from providing the same or similar services to other physicians whereas the physician may want an exclusive arrangement with the hospital.

Compensation

With regard to the compensation to be provided to the hospital, various alternatives exist. For example, the hospital may be compensated on a cost-plus basis equal to the total cost to the hospital for providing the services plus some fixed or variable figure. A typical monthly compensation provision formulated on a cost-plus basis is as follows:

> *Monthly compensation.* For the first 12 months of the term of this Agreement, compensation from the Physician to the Hospital shall be a total of $_____, which the Hospital represents to be its best estimate of its costs of rendering such services plus 15%, payable by the Physician in 12 equal monthly installments of _____ on the first day of each month.
>
> For the next following 12 months of the term of this Agreement, compensation from the Physician to the Hospital shall be a total of $ _____, which the Hospital represents to be its best estimate of its costs of rendering services plus 15%, payable by the Physician in 12 equal monthly installments of _____ on the first day of each month.
>
> For each month after the initial 24 months of this Agreement, the Physician shall pay to the Hospital monthly, on the first day of each month, an amount equal to 115% of the sum set forth on the month-to-month budget as the cost of services provided by the Hospital during that month.

Such a compensation provision requires that the following cost-accounting and adjustment provision be included in the agreement:

Cost accountings and adjustments. Within ninety (90) days after the end of each year of this Agreement, commencing with the year ending _____ , and within ninety (90) days after termination of this Agreement, an annual cost accounting shall be prepared at the Hospital's expense of the actual costs incurred by the Hospital in providing the services required under this Agreement during the year just completed or during the period since completion of the last annual cost accounting.

If sums paid by the Physician to the Hospital exceed one hundred fifteen percent (115%) of the Hospital's actual cost of providing services to the Physician, the Hospital shall reimburse the Physician in cash, within thirty (30) days after notice of completion of the annual cost accounting, an amount equal to one hundred percent (100%) of the difference. If sums paid by the Physician to the Hospital are less than one hundred fifteen percent (115%) of the Hospital's actual cost, the Physician shall pay in cash an amount equal to one hundred percent (100%) of the difference to the Hospital within thirty (30) days after notice of completion of the annual cost accounting. Notice of completion of the annual cost accounting shall include a copy of the calculations and supporting data for any reimbursement or payment required by this Section. The Physician shall have thirty (30) days after receipt of the annual cost-accounting report to object to or dispute any calculation or data contained therein by written notice to the Hospital. If the Physician fails so to object, the physician shall be deemed to have accepted the report. If the Physician does so object, the parties shall attempt to resolve their dispute within the next following thirty (30) days, after which time, if there is no resolution, either party may submit the dispute to arbitration in accordance with Section _____ of this Agreement.

The compensation mechanism may also be based on a percentage of gross or net income to the physician or on a per hour or per project basis. Another alternative is for the hospital to be retained on a straight salary basis, with the salary payable on a monthly basis.

In preparing any compensation provision, you should be mindful of the various legal issues applicable to the relationship. See chapter 5 for a detailed description of the relevant legal issues.

Budget for Services

The agreement may include a provision requiring the creation of a budget for services to be provided. Such a provision may take the following form:

Budget for services. The services to be provided by the Hospital shall be described in a month-to-month budget, prepared annually by the

Hospital and, upon approval by the Physician, attached to this Agreement as consecutively numbered riders. Each budget shall include an estimate of the cost of each service to be provided by the Hospital. Such costs shall be estimated by the Hospital to include 100% of the direct and indirect costs incurred by the Hospital in providing the services to the Physician. The Hospital shall submit each annual budget to the Physician for review and approval at least sixty days prior to the end of each year of the Hospital preceding the year for which the budget will be applicable. The Physician may accept or reject for good cause, or suggest modifications to any such budget or any line item thereof. If the final budget is not accepted by both parties prior to the beginning of the year to which it is to apply, the Agreement shall terminate at the end of the preceding year.

Confidentiality of Proprietary Information

In connection with the provision of services by the hospital to the physician, the hospital may wish to prohibit the physician from using certain methods, procedures, and other information developed by the hospital and made available to the physician. It may be advisable to include a confidentiality provision in the agreement in the following form:

Confidentiality of proprietary information. In the course of the relationship created pursuant to this Agreement, the Physician will have access to certain methods, operations, trade secrets, processes, data, procedures, publications, materials, documents, know-how, techniques, forms, trade information, and confidential or other proprietary information (collectively referred to as "Proprietary Information") regarding the operations of the Hospital. The Physician shall maintain all such Proprietary Information in strict secrecy and shall not, directly or indirectly, disclose or divulge such information to any third parties, except as may be necessary for the discharge of the obligations of the Physician hereunder. The Physician shall not directly or indirectly take or use Proprietary Information for the Physician's purposes or the purposes of others at any time during or after the term of this Agreement except as may be necessary for the discharge of the Physician's obligations hereunder. The Physician shall not remove, retain, or copy, without the express prior written consent of the Hospital, any Proprietary Information of any type or description. Upon termination of this Agreement for any reason, the Physician shall immediately return and restore to the Hospital Proprietary Information belonging to the Hospital and all originals or copies of documents in whatever form relating to Proprietary Information. The Hospital is hereby specifically made a third-party beneficiary of this section with the power to enforce the provisions hereof. The Physician recognizes that a breach of this section cannot be adequately compensated in money damages and therefore agrees that injunctive relief shall be available to the Hospital.

Joint Venture Arrangements

A joint venture arrangement involves a single-purpose or multipurpose joint venture between the hospital and the physician for the purpose of owning and operating clinical programs such as diagnostic imaging centers, surgery centers, or other outpatient facilities. The purpose of the joint venture is to enhance the clinical aspects of a physician's practice while at the same time creating an economic interdependence between the hospital and the physician through shared investment.

This type of arrangement involves the creation of either a partnership or a corporation. If a partnership is formed, a general or limited partnership agreement needs to be prepared to spell out, among other things, the duties and responsibilities of the partners and the distribution of profits and losses. A provision governing the transferability of interest in the partnership is advisable. If the corporate form is more desirable, articles of incorporation, bylaws and various organizational documents need to be prepared to govern the day-to-day operations of the corporation. Again, a provision addressing the transferability of the interest should be included in the corporate bylaws.

Medical Directorships (or Consultancies)

The category of medical directorships (or consultancies) covers a number of different arrangements between the hospital and the physician, all of which pertain to the management of clinical departments or services. For example, the physician could serve either as an employee of or independent contractor to the hospital and could be responsible for the clinical aspects of a hospital department or service, the administrative aspects, or both.

Responsibilities of the Medical Director

The agreement should delineate the responsibilities delegated to the medical director and may take the following form:

> *Responsibilities of the medical director.* As Medical Director, the Physician shall be responsible generally for the supervision and management of the overall professional and clinical aspects of care rendered by the Hospital and its employees and for the medico-administrative operations of the _____ Department. The Physician's responsibilities as Medical Director shall include but not be limited to the following:

a. Professional and administrative direction and supervision of, and accountability to, the Hospital with respect to all professional and clinical services provided by the _____ Department;

b. Review and evaluation of the efficacy, validity, and appropriateness of therapeutic techniques employed, and of the quality of health care services provided, by the _____ Department;

c. Review and evaluation of the Hospital's compliance with applicable laws and regulations of federal, state, and local governments and with applicable standards for licensure and accreditation;

d. Review and evaluation of medical equipment used by the _____ Department for safety and therapeutic value;

e. Participation with the Hospital in the development of annual capital and operating budgets of the _____ Department;

f. Participation with the Hospital in the development of appropriate policies and procedures for patient care in the _____ Department;

g. Coordination of medical care rendered by the _____ Department and maintenance of effective liaison with attending physicians;

h. Supervision of the nursing and nonprofessional support staffs of the _____ Department;

i. Acquisition and maintenance of medical equipment for the _____ Department in accordance with annual capital and operating budgets; and

j. Performance of all other duties of the Physician set forth in this Agreement and all other duties required for the efficient and safe operation of the _____ Department.

Another important provision to be included in the agreement involves the allocation of time by the medical director in connection with the services and responsibilities delegated to this physician. Sample provisions include the following:

Allocation of time. The Physician shall devote a minimum of _____ (_____) hours per week to the fulfillment of the duties of Medical Director as provided hereunder, and so much additional time as shall be necessary and appropriate in keeping with the objective of providing high-quality professional and clinical services to the _____ Department. Subject to the foregoing and to his or her patient care responsibilities, nothing contained in this Section shall be construed as prohibiting the Physician from carrying on or devoting substantial time to other activities in which he or she may engage, including without limitation the practice of medicine, provided, however, that the Physician shall not serve as medical director of any other facility or entity or provide medical services to patients except in connection with the provision of services pursuant to this Agreement.

Coverage. During the term of this Agreement, the Physician and such Practitioners as are approved by the Hospital pursuant to subparagraph _____ below shall provide the Services to patients during the business hours of the Hospital and shall supply on-call services for nonbusiness hours, emergencies, weekends, and holidays. The Physician and/or sufficient Practitioners shall be available at all times during normal business hours for direct consultation with attending physicians and patients. The Physician acknowledges that the patient load in the Department is particularly heavy in the early morning, the noon hour, and the late afternoon. In consideration of the foregoing, the Physician shall develop a schedule, agreed upon by the Physician and the Hospital (the "Schedule"), for the provision of Services that indicates an adequate number of Practitioners, including the Physician, who will be on site and on call during business hours and nonbusiness hours. Neither the Physician nor any Practitioner shall be absent from the Department during his or her scheduled days for the provision of services, as set forth on the Schedule then in effect, for more than forty-two (42) calendar days during any year of this Agreement. The foregoing limitation shall apply to an absence for any reason, including but not limited to vacation, holidays, illness, or attendance at seminars or continuing education programs, but excluding absences for teaching responsibilities approved by the Hospital.

Utilization of Other Practitioners

The agreement should also address whether the physician appointed as medical director (or consultant) may engage the services of other practitioners in order to fulfill the obligations under the agreement. If the parties agree that the physician may engage the services of other physicians, the provision may take the following form:

Practitioners. The Physician hereby warrants that he or she has furnished a complete and accurate copy of the agreement that he or she intends to utilize to engage Practitioners to provide Services in connection with this Agreement. In addition, copies of all executed agreements between the Physician and any such Practitioners relating to the provision of Services shall be furnished to the Hospital prior to the effective date thereof to enable the Hospital to determine that the provisions thereof are consistent with the terms of this Agreement. No such agreement shall have any force or effect prior to review and approval by the Hospital. All designations of Practitioners to perform Services shall be subject to the prior written approval of the Hospital. If the Hospital determines that the Practitioners fail to meet the requirements of Section _____ of this Agreement, then such Practitioners shall not be entitled to perform Services on behalf of the Physician. The Physician shall give the Hospital at least thirty (30) days' prior written notice of and consult with the Hospital regarding the addition or termination of any Practitioner. The authority of each Practitioner to perform the Services under this Agreement shall be subject to compliance by each Practitioner with the requirements for Practitioners set forth in this Agreement.

If the responsibilities delegated to the physician involve the preparation of records and reports, the hospital should include a provision requiring the physician and each practitioner providing services to the hospital to maintain customary medical records and written reports, which remain the property of the hospital. In addition, the hospital may deem it appropriate to require the physician and each practitioner to cooperate with and assist members of the medical staff of the hospital in the preparation of clinical reports for publication and to use their best efforts to elevate the standing of the medical staff in the relevant field by publication of unusual or interesting studies made in the department.

It may be also appropriate to require the physician and all practitioners to comply with the rules, regulations, policies, and procedures of the hospital and to participate in the hospital's quality assurance program. In addition, the hospital may also require the physician and other practitioners engaged by the physician to maintain medical staff privileges with the hospital. If such a provision is included in the agreement, the termination clause may be triggered upon the cessation of all privileges of the physician or other practitioners at the hospital.

Conversely, the medical staff privileges of the physician may be tied to the continuance of the contractual arrangement between the hospital and physician in those arrangements where the physician is granted the exclusive right to operate the department. A detailed discussion of the legal and political ramifications of such an arrangement is beyond the scope of this chapter, and state law should be reviewed to determine if such a provision is enforceable. For example, under California law, closed staffs adopted by a hospital whereby the hospital grants a physician the exclusive right to operate the department under a contractual arrangement have been upheld as a reasonable exercise of the hospital's powers to adopt rules and regulations for operating the hospital.[1] In addition, the *Accreditation Manual for Hospitals* allows a hospital to tie continued medical staff membership to the continuance of a contractual arrangement in the case of a physician active in administrative capacities in the hospital.[2]

Service Site

The agreement should clearly set forth the location of the services to be provided by the physician on behalf of the hospital. For example, will the physician be providing the services in the hospital, in an outpatient department located in another facility, or in a mobile unit or any other facility the hospital desires? The agreement should also contain a description of the facilities and equipment provided to the physician by the hospital, such as access to the premises, equipment and supplies for providing the services at the premises, utilities, nonmedical personnel, ancillary and support services, and the like.

Compensation

Finally, the agreement must address the issue of compensation to the physician. For example, the compensation for services rendered can be by salary or stipend and can be fixed or tied to some floating economic measure such as the gross operational revenue of the program. One example of a compensation mechanism that may be included in a typical medical director agreement is as follows:

> *Compensation.* The Physician shall at all times maintain a schedule of professional fees for the Services rendered in the Department that is reasonable and customary with respect to professional fees for similar services rendered to patients in the community. The fee schedule and all amendments and restatements thereof shall be subject to the prior approval of the Hospital. The schedule approved by the Hospital to be placed in effect at the commencement of this Agreement is attached to this Agreement as Exhibit "_____." If at any time the Hospital reasonably determines that the fee schedule then in effect does not reflect the reasonable and customary charges in the community, it shall so advise the Physician, and the Physician shall revise the fee schedule accordingly. The Physician shall amend the fee schedule in proportion to any increase or decrease in the Hospital's fee schedule. The Physician may amend the fee schedule otherwise only with the prior approval of the Hospital. If at any time the Hospital and the Physician cannot agree on a revision to the schedule of professional fees, the dispute shall, on written request of one party served on the other, be submitted to arbitration in accordance with Section _____ of this Agreement.

Agreements for the Acquisition of Physician Practices

A hospital can structure its acquired physician practices in myriad ways, as set forth in chapter 4. This section discusses the agreements to be developed in the following key categories:

- Hospital assists a legally independent physician group in its acquisition of practices.
- Hospital acquires nonclinical aspects of a physician's practice and leases them back to the practitioner.
- Hospital acquires clinical and nonclinical aspects of the practice.

Assisting a Legally Independent Physician Group in Its Acquisition of Practices

As discussed in chapter 4, an agreement whereby the hospital assists a legally independent physician group in its acquisition of practices is typified by an existing single-specialty or multispecialty group practice that approaches the hospital for assistance in developing a series of satellites through practice acquisitions. Alternatively, several physicians may desire to start up a fully integrated group by combining their practices and acquiring other practices.

The hospital may be of assistance in either of these alternatives by providing facilities, such as satellite practice sites, or by purchasing or leasing new sites or upgrading facilities, then equipping and leasing such sites to the physician group or making such sites available through another form of use arrangement. The relationship between the hospital and the physician may take the form of a contractual agreement whereby the hospital leases property it owns to the physician; or alternatively, if the hospital is leasing the premises, the hospital subleases the property to the physician. The hospital could also sell the property, whether real or personal, to the physician under a standard purchase and sale agreement or could assist the physician in purchasing the property. This assistance could take the form of lending money to the physician, guaranteeing debt obligations incurred by the physician, or contributing capital to the project on a shared investment basis.

Leased Equipment

The hospital may offer its assistance by leasing equipment it owns (or leases) to the physician under a standard equipment lease. Such an agreement should include a provision describing in detail the equipment to be leased to the physician. The description may be included in the body of the agreement or may be described in an exhibit attached to the agreement.

The rent payable to the hospital could be based on the gross income derived by the physician from the use and operation of the equipment less all reasonable expenses to operate the equipment and reasonable reserves determined by the physician for contingencies and anticipated obligations. Alternatively, the rent could be based on a modified gross or modified net figure, could be the hospital's cost of owning the equipment plus some fixed percentage, or could be a fixed monthly fee. In addition to the payment of rent, the agreement should specify whether the hospital or the physician is required to pay taxes and other charges arising in connection with the equipment, including licensing, real or personal property, gross receipts, or other taxes due on the equipment. The agreement also should address the maintenance and repairs of the equipment and should specify the party responsible for keeping the equipment in good repair. Typically, the physician, as lessee, would be required to maintain maintenance agreements and would otherwise take responsibility for keeping the equipment in good working order.

The specific location where the equipment will be housed should be specified in the agreement. If the physician is authorized to relocate the equipment to other premises, the agreement should include provisions governing the removal, relocation, and installation of the equipment at the new premises.

A standard warranty disclaimer provision, such as that which follows, should be included in the agreement:

> *Warranty disclaimer.* Except as otherwise expressly provided in this Agreement, the Hospital has made and makes no representations or warranties, either expressed or implied, and shall not, by virtue of having leased the equipment covered by this Agreement, be deemed to have made any representation or warranty as to the title, merchantability, fitness, design, or condition of the equipment, or the quality of the material or workmanship in the equipment, for any particular purpose or as to the conformity of the equipment to specifications or purchase order or as to its design, delivery, installation, or operation.

Title to the equipment should remain with the hospital, and a provision should be included that specifically reserves title to the hospital. If the equipment involves computer hardware and/or software and the physician might be developing software in connection with the use of the equipment, the ownership of this software should be addressed. An example of a provision reserving title to the hospital follows:

> *Development and ownership.* The Physician shall have the right, in his or her own discretion, to modify independently the software portions of the equipment for his or her own purpose and use, provided that the Physician does not disclose or distribute any part of such software except as permitted by the Hospital. All software programs developed hereunder are proprietary to the Hospital, and title thereto shall remain in the Hospital. All applicable rights to patents, copyrights, trademarks, and trade secrets in such software are and shall remain in the Hospital.

If the hospital is leasing computer software, the agreement should contain a provision whereby the hospital grants to the physician a license to use the software:

Licenses. The Hospital grants to the Physician a nonexclusive, nontransferable license to use such software for the Physician's use on the equipment and to sublicense such software to third parties in accordance with a standard written license agreement approved by the Hospital between such third parties and the Physician or the Hospital. Each such agreement or sublicense with the third parties shall expressly give the Hospital the right to enforce the terms of such a standard software license agreement against the third parties and shall state that the software is the proprietary property of the Hospital.

Infringement. The Physician will at his or her own expense defend, indemnify, and hold harmless the Hospital in connection with any action based on a claim that any aspect of software developed by the Physician hereunder infringes any patents, copyrights, licenses, or trade secrets of others.

Other Provisions

An agreement whereby the hospital assists a legally independent physician group in its acquisition of practices may include other provisions as well. For example, a standard provision on confidentiality of proprietary information is strongly recommended. See the example of such a provision earlier in this chapter.

In addition, the hospital may want to grant the physician an option to purchase the equipment upon termination of the agreement. Such a provision should state in detail the terms and conditions relating to the physician's right to purchase the equipment.

Hospital assistance also can take the form of administrative and clinical support services, which was discussed earlier in this chapter, or the complete management of a physician's practice under a turnkey management agreement, which is discussed in the following section.

Acquiring the Nonclinical Aspects of a Physician's Practice and Leasing Them Back to the Physician

An arrangement in which the hospital acquires the nonclinical aspects of a physician's practice involves the transfer to the hospital under a purchase and sale agreement of selected assets and liabilities of the physician. The physician retains the clinical aspects of the practice as well as the legal form of doing business. Once transferred, the assets may be leased back to the physician under a lease agreement coupled with a management and administrative services agreement.

To accomplish this arrangement, the hospital and physician should enter into a standard purchase and sale-of-assets agreement. The agreement includes, among other things, the following provisions:

- A description of all assets to be purchased and liabilities to be assumed by the hospital
- The amount of the purchase price and the payment terms
- A description of the security for payment of the purchase price
- Standard representations and warranties of the physician

If the physician desires to lease the assets purchased by the hospital, the parties should also enter into standard lease agreements (see the earlier discussion on leased equipment). The hospital may also want to provide certain administrative and clinical support services (see the discussion at the beginning of this chapter).

The physician may decide to delegate all management responsibilities associated with the nonclinical aspects of his or her practice to the hospital and retain responsibility only for the clinical aspects of the practice. Such an arrangement involves the development of a *turnkey management agreement* between the hospital and the physician. The agreement involves the use by the physician of certain space, equipment, furnishings, and other property for the physician's use in connection with his or her practice of medicine and the provision by the hospital to the physician of services and personnel relating to the operation, management, supervision, and administration of the nonmedical aspects of the physician's practice, as well as business planning and development support.

With regard to the facility made available to the physician, the turnkey management agreement should include a provision describing the real and personal property subject to use by the physician. Oftentimes, this description is the same as the description contained in the asset purchase agreement entered into between the hospital and the physician, under which the physician sells the nonclinical aspects of his or her practice to the hospital. Other standard provisions relating to the use of real and personal property by the physician include a description of the obligations of the hospital to maintain and repair the property, an acknowledgment by the physician that the hospital makes no express or implied warranties or representations with regard to the real or personal property, a statement of the rights and liabilities of the physician and the hospital in the event the real property is destroyed, and a statement that the title to the personal property remains with the hospital.

Additional, Substitute, or Replacement Equipment

Oftentimes, a physician may request the hospital to replace or substitute personal property or to provide additional equipment during the term of the turnkey management agreement. A provision should be included in the agreement that specifies the parties' rights and liabilities in such an event:

Additional, substitute, or replacement equipment. In the event the Physician requests the Hospital to replace or substitute any item of Equipment or to provide additional equipment during the term hereof, the Hospital shall in its reasonable discretion determine whether such equipment is considered reasonable and necessary equipment by other comparable physician practices located in _____ area. If the Hospital determines that such Equipment is reasonable and necessary, it shall endeavor to locate a suitable source for such Equipment at a reasonable price and to acquire and provide the use of such Equipment to the Physician pursuant to the terms and conditions hereof, provided, however, that the Hospital shall be entitled to a reasonable adjustment to the ceiling of expenses provided for in Section _____ hereunder to cover any increase in its costs of performance attributable to such additional, substitute, or replacement equipment. Nothing contained herein shall prevent or prohibit the Physician from purchasing for his or her own account and at his or her own expense such equipment as the Hospital determines is not reasonable and necessary hereunder, provided that the Physician complies at his or her own cost and expense with all applicable governmental laws, ordinances, or regulations and the installation and maintenance does not require any alteration, addition, or improvement of the Facility. At the expiration or termination of this agreement, the Physician shall have the right to remove his or her equipment, provided the Physician is not in default at the time of removal and provided further that he or she shall, at the time of removal of such equipment, repair in a good and workmanlike manner any damage caused by installation or removal thereof. For purposes of this agreement, any additional, substitute, or replacement equipment acquired by the Hospital shall be deemed included in and a part of the Equipment, as such term is used herein.

Management and Administrative Services

Another aspect of the turnkey management agreement involves the management and administrative services to be provided by the hospital to the physician. A typical provision states that the physician engages the hospital to serve as the physician's exclusive manager and administrator of the nonmedical aspects of his or her practice. It is appropriate to require the hospital to prepare and deliver to the physician an annual budget that sets out major operating objectives and anticipated revenues, expenses, and cash flows respecting the physician's practice at the facility.

Billing and Collection

Another provision typically found in turnkey management agreements involves the billing and collection services provided by the hospital to the physician:

Billing and collection. The Hospital shall furnish to the Physician all necessary billing and collection services respecting medical services rendered by the Physician at the Facility commencing on the effective date of this Agreement. Without limiting the generality of the foregoing, the Hospital shall train on-site personnel to the extent necessary to provide for the orderly billing of accounts receivable. The Hospital and the Physician shall reasonably agree upon accounts receivable to be assigned to collection agencies prior to any such assignment.

Deposit and disbursement of funds. The Hospital shall deposit in such bank accounts as the Hospital shall designate on behalf of the Physician all receipts and monies from the operation of the practice collected by the Hospital. During the term of this Agreement, the Hospital shall have the authority to write checks against or otherwise withdraw funds deposited in the Physician's bank account for the purposes described in this Agreement. Furthermore, the Hospital shall have the authority to commingle all such receipts and monies collected or received on behalf of any or all physicians providing medical services at the facility pursuant to the terms of turnkey management agreements entered into with the Hospital. The Hospital agrees to assume all risks and liabilities relating to the improper use of any such bank accounts and agrees to hold the Physician harmless with respect thereto.

Marketing and Business Development

Other services to be provided by the hospital under a turnkey management agreement include marketing and business development. Such a provision obligates the hospital to provide such marketing services for the physician's medical practice as may be submitted to and reviewed and approved by the physician. All such marketing must be in compliance with applicable laws and regulations governing the use of advertising by physicians in the state where the physician's practice is located. The hospital may also make recommendations and assist the physician in developing patient education materials and programs or changes in the scope of services offered by the physician. In addition, the hospital may provide business development support and consultation to the physician as needed by the physician from time to time.

Personnel

A turnkey management agreement should address the issue of personnel to satisfy and perform the obligations of the hospital under the agreement. For example, the hospital may retain the right to employ and otherwise engage all personnel it deems necessary and at its sole cost and expense to satisfy and perform its obligations under the agreement. As to "on-site personnel," which could be defined as all persons whose primary place of work is at the physician's practice, the hospital may be required to employ, at its cost and expense, such on-site personnel consisting of the number of registered nurses, medical assistants, and other categories of service providers as reasonably agreed upon by the hospital and the physician as necessary and beneficial in the operation of the physician's practice. The hospital should retain the sole and exclusive responsibility of hiring, discharging, and supervising all nonphysician personnel engaged in nonmedical functions who are provided to the physician pursuant to the agreement. In states where the corporate practice of medicine doctrine may be applicable (see chapter 5), the physician is required to retain sole responsibility for the supervision, hiring, or discharge of all personnel engaged in connection with all medical functions of the physician's practice.

Physician's Obligations

Typically, the turnkey management agreement contains a detailed discussion of the physician's obligations under the agreement. The physician should be required to comply with all laws, regulations, and ethical and professional standards applicable to the professional practice of medicine and should be required to maintain an active medical staff status with the hospital. The physician should also be required to devote his full-time abilities and attention to his practice during the term of the agreement.

Covenant Not to Compete

Of vital importance is determining whether the turnkey management agreement should include a covenant-not-to-compete clause. An analysis of the applicable state law governing the agreement needs to be conducted to determine whether the state would uphold a provision prohibiting the physician from rendering medical services similar to those provided by the physician at the facility during the term of the agreement and, upon termination of the agreement, at a location other than the one managed by the hospital. In states that would strike down the validity of such a provision, a hospital may at least want to prohibit a physician from using confidential and proprietary information both during the term of the agreement and after its termination (see the sample confidentiality provision earlier in this chapter).

An example of a typical covenant-not-to-compete provision follows:

Covenant not to compete. Except as otherwise provided below,
   a. during the term of this Agreement,
   b. until seven (7) years from the effective date of this Agreement if it is terminated during its initial five (5) year term, and

c. for an additional two (2) year period following any subsequent termination of this Agreement, the Physician shall not, directly or indirectly, own an interest in, operate, join, control, participate in, or be connected in any manner with any corporation, partnership, proprietorship, firm, association, person, or entity providing medical services similar to the care to be provided by the Physician in the Practice and located within _____ County, _____. This covenant shall be limited to one (1) year following any election by the Hospital not to renew this Agreement and shall not apply following any termination of this Agreement pursuant to Section _____ or for cause by the Physician. This covenant shall not be construed to prohibit the Physician from performing professional medical services for patients as part of the Practice at hospitals other than the Hospital, provided, however, that the Physician agrees that he or she shall maintain his or her primary active staff membership at the Hospital and, to the extent practicable and as consistent with the principles of sound medical practice and the desires of individual patients, the Physician shall refer patients to other physicians and specialists who maintain staff membership at the Hospital.

The parties acknowledge that the geographic and practice restrictions under this Agreement and the period of such restrictions are reasonable and necessary for the adequate protection of the Hospital with respect to the transactions contemplated by this Agreement. The Physician agrees that a violation of any of the terms or conditions of this Section will cause irreparable harm and injury to the Hospital, which is extremely difficult or impossible to ascertain, and that any remedy at law for breach thereof will be inadequate. Accordingly, the Hospital shall be entitled, as a matter of course and in addition to any other rights or remedies, to an injunction issued out of any court of competent jurisdiction enjoining or restraining the Physician from continuing to do any act or commit any violation or threatened violation of this Section, and the Physician hereby consents to the issuance of such injunction or restraining order.

Compensation

In an arrangement where the nonmedical aspects of a physician's practice are managed by the hospital, including billing and collection services, it is appropriate to include a provision governing the compensation due the physician for the provision of medical services rendered at the facility. The physician may be compensated from the gross revenues of the practice in the form of a base compensation and receive additional compensation in the form of bonus compensation. Base compensation may equal a percentage of a specified sum. The specified sum can be adjusted annually after a determination of the net income earned from the physician's practice during the previous year. The physician could be eligible for bonus compensation in the event the net income is greater than the total amount paid to the physician as base compensation.

The compensation due the hospital must also be addressed in the turnkey management agreement. The hospital may receive an amount equal to the gross revenues collected by or on behalf of the physician relating to the physician's practice remaining after the hospital pays all applicable costs and expenses of the practice described in the agreement and pays the amounts due the physician as compensation. Such a fee could be payable to the hospital on a monthly basis, and the hospital could retain a right to withdraw amounts from the physician's bank accounts to the extent necessary to pay the monthly management fee.

Acquiring Clinical and Nonclinical Aspects of the Practice

When both the clinical and nonclinical aspects of a physician's practice are transferred to a hospital, the physician ceases his or her current legal structure of practice and becomes either an employee or independent contractor of the hospital or its affiliate.

As was discussed in chapter 4, the acquisition of the practice may be accomplished according to the single-tiered approach, under which the physician transfers his or her entire practice and becomes a professional employee of the hospital or its affiliate or provides services in the new practice setting as an independent contractor. Alternatively, the acquisition may be accomplished under the two-tiered approach, which involves the complete sale and transfer of the practice but bifurcates the nonclinical aspects from the clinical portion of the practice, with the former going to the hospital or its affiliate and the latter going to a related group practice (RGP).

Two-Tiered Approach

If the approach is two tiered, the acquisition of the nonclinical aspects of the physician's practice is accomplished in accordance with the agreements discussed in the previous section on turnkey management agreements. The acquisition of the clinical aspects of the practice could be accomplished by merging the physician's practice with that of the RGP or by the physician's selling his or her medical practice to the RGP. In return, the physician could receive shares of stock in the RGP or could be paid the fair market value of his or her practice. In addition, the physician could be required to enter into an employment or independent contract agreement with the RGP to perform full-time professional medical services for the RGP.

A physician's practice may be combined with the RGP pursuant to a merger agreement with the RGP. The agreement should provide that the RGP is the surviving corporation and the physician's practice is the disappearing entity. As the surviving corporation, the RGP succeeds to all the assets and liabilities of the disappearing entity, including all agreements to which the entity is a party, and the RGP becomes the employer of all physician employees of the entity. The merger should be structured so as to comply with the relevant state law governing the transaction.

If either the RGP or the physician deems it inappropriate to combine the practices pursuant to the merger agreement, the parties may enter into a transfer agreement pursuant to which the physician agrees to transfer certain tangible and intangible property, including medical records, used in the physician's practice. The physician also agrees to assign or cause to be assigned to the RGP certain agreements to which the physician is a party.

In either event, the physician may continue providing medical services by entering into an employment or independent contractual arrangement with the RGP. Under an employment agreement, the physician agrees to conduct all of his or her medical practice through the RGP and not perform medical services for profit either individually or for another person or organization (see the earlier discussion regarding the applicability and enforceability of a covenant-not-to-compete provision). The facilities, services, and benefits provided by the RGP should also be set forth in the employment agreement.

Compensation

The compensation mechanism can be structured in a variety of ways: The physician can receive a straight salary, an amount per hour, a percentage or modified percentage of gross or net income associated with the physician's practice, or a salary based on the collections of the RGP attributable to the physician's services less an amount attributable to certain items of overhead. For example, the collections of the RGP attributable to the physician's services could be reduced by:

- A percentage attributable to a corporate reserve account and held for payment of contingency fees
- The physician's share of common corporate expenses
- A percentage of the receipts allocated to a common pool of funds distributed equally to all physicians who provide professional services to or on behalf of the RGP
- The cost of certain services, personnel, facilities, and benefits specifically applicable to the physician

An independent contractual relationship is similar to the employment relationship except that the physician has more mobility to practice outside the RGP setting and is not entitled to fringe benefits otherwise granted to a physician employee.

Conclusion

In any transaction involving the acquisition or enhancement of a physician's practice, innumerable duties and responsibilities of the parties must be spelled out clearly in appropriate contracts. These could include the transfer of assets, the provision of administrative services by the hospital to the physician, management agreements, and the duties and responsibilities of the physician to provide defined clinical and perhaps administrative services as well. The terms and conditions of these responsibilities must be clearly understood by the parties, and there is no substitute for written contracts that spell out such responsibilities. Although many of the key features that are likely to be encountered in such agreements were discussed in this chapter, given the variety of possibilities it is imperative that the written agreements be precisely tailored to fit the specific circumstances.

Notes

1. *Blank v. Palo Alto–Stanford Hospital Center,* 234 *Cal.2d* 377 (1965); *Centeno v. Roseville Community Hospital,* 107 *Cal.3d* 62 (1979).

2. Joint Commission on Accreditation of Healthcare Organizations. *Accreditation Manual for Hospitals.* Chicago: JCAHO, 1987. See Standard MS.1, Required Characteristics MS.1.2.3.1.14; Standard MS.4, Required Characteristics MS.4.2.12.

Chapter 9

Making the Acquisition Work

Philip A. Newbold and Rex S. Levering

To complete the process of negotiation and execute a final agreement are major accomplishments. By now your transaction has survived the scrutiny and due diligence of hospital administrators, accountants, lawyers, outside practice consultants, physicians, and board members. But once the agreement is signed, you need to call in an entirely new team to set up corporate systems and oversee the management of the practice. Successful acquisitions programs include a broad representation of operations and systems people in the initial development and negotiating team to ensure a smooth transition after the acquisition and to provide some continuity of management and leadership.

In terms of corporate accounting, purchasing, information processing, corporate marketing, and the like, the newly acquired practice may no longer be operated as a partnership or professional corporation but, instead, as an operating unit of a large corporate system. Anxiety and conflict are the natural products of such a transition unless the managers are exceptionally astute in stabilizing and strengthening the relationship in the early months after the deal closes. Before acquiring your first medical practice, consider the pitfalls of "corporatizing" the physician's office. Based on nearly a decade of experience, the authors have found that many seasoned deal makers rule out connecting managed practices to many corporate or acute hospital operating systems.

Avoiding Corporatization

The road map for the hospital's course of action after the closing is the set of agreements reached during the courtship and negotiation process.

Effective practice managers have learned to limit their changes to only the most critical items, especially during the first year of the "marriage." Changes that will be necessary are those the physician expects as a result of the negotiation process and those brought about by uncharted crisis. For example, the hospital and physician may have agreed to replace the "senior" office manager immediately after the deal closes. Or the hospital may have an unexpected need for capital to acquire a new office location and may need to sell the real estate of the newly acquired practice.

But in the absence of compelling reasons, you should heed the oft-cited advice: "If it's not broken, don't fix it." Experienced operators report some "dos and don'ts" for newcomers to practice management:

- Changes to avoid in the transition period (as long as there is no crisis)
  - Major changes in office hours, physician staffing, and employee staffing
  - Change in practice location
  - Radical change in the billing, receivables, or collection systems
  - Trading the current office computer for the hospital's information system or computer network
- Most successful innovations during the transition period
  - New tools for communicating with current or prospective patients, including newsletters, direct-mail pieces, and thank-you notes
  - Wellness and education programs newly introduced in the physician's office
  - Customer relations skills introduced to the office staff as well as ongoing patient-satisfaction measurement devices and problem-solving systems

Managing the Thriving Practice

Smart operators think long and hard before imposing the hospital's corporate systems on a thriving practice, regardless of the strategic plan or corporate policy. This excludes, of course, cash controls, tracking systems, and monitoring of revenues, expenses, patient referrals, and visits. All these controls are routine and basic essentials in acquiring any business, large or small. At the level of corporate accounting, the shift from cash accounting to an accrual accounting system, if necessary, can be accomplished with little or no impact on daily routines of practice employees.

Community and Patient Notification

One typical issue that is sensitive and does need good planning and careful consideration is how to notify the community of the new ownership or new relationship. Many marketers want to "brand name" the private practice with new signage that identifies the practice as "affiliated with ABC Hospital." Care should be taken to ensure that this message results in an overall positive, long-term effect on the practice and does not confuse the public or potential referring physicians as to what the affiliation really means.

Another issue is the notification of past and present patients as to the new ownership or economic relationship. Usually a letter to all patients explaining the new relationship and a listing of the benefits and advantages is useful and effective. Figure 9.1 is an example of a letter that is both informative and helpful in sustaining and building the newly acquired private practice.

The Role of the Champion

When practice employees go onto the system "payroll," staff attitudes are ripe for turning sour—first toward the corporation and then toward the physician who "sold out." Consider assigning a recognized, clearly identified champion from within the organization to assist a newly acquired practice. Characteristics of this champion include high credibility with employees and physicians, previous experience, time to devote to the practice, and an empathetic style of interpersonal skills. For example, after five years of hospital management experience, one successful champion in the north-central United States saw a new career opportunity in heading up the newly formed practice management subsidiary. Another champion had a long and successful history as an urban medical center's director of outreach education and sales programs targeted at rural communities. This individual was already well known and liked by physicians and hospital administrators throughout the region.

High on the champion's list of priorities is keeping attitudes within the practice healthy while serving as a direct link between the physician's staff and top-level management. The champion's ultimate challenge is to overcome the "we" versus "they" mentality that may creep into the morale of any acquired business. But his or her most important roles are (1) fostering the entrepreneurial spirit of the practice and keeping the sense of accountability for high standards of patient service within the office itself; and (2) defending the practice against the "system builders" who want to replace private practice accountability with corporatization of the practice network. Examples of system builders include the personnel administrator intent on making personnel practices uniform throughout the system or the department of information systems determined to replace the freestanding (but well-functioning) physician office computer with the corporation's integrated system. All too often, the hospital's system is simply less effective for medical practice applications.

Figure 9.1. Sample Letter Announcing a Practice Acquisition to Patients

---

JOHN R. DOE, M.D., F.A.A.F.P.
Family Practice

2100 Sharewood Court
Elsewhere, Ohio   44000

July 1, 1988

Dear Patient:

I am writing to you to share our plans for moving into an exciting new family practice affiliation with additional board-certified family physicians. Each physician and nurse practitioner will continue seeing all our own private patients just as we do now. The major advantage for you will be immediate accessibility to an affiliated physician when we are not available. And, for your convenience, we will be able to extend our appointment hours into some evenings and weekends when we are fully staffed.

This summer we will move our practices into a comprehensive new clinical facility now under construction near the intersection of Maywood Avenue and Heritage Drive. Operated in cooperation with Elsewhere Medical Center, the new facility will enable us to provide our patients with more support services, including expanded laboratory, X-ray, and other diagnostic capabilities.

Wishing you good health,

John R. Doe, M.D.,
   and Staff

Bookkeeping and Other Management Practices

The bookkeeping and other management practices of some private practices are quite different from those of the hospital and can present some challenging problems. Whether these management practices are termed "loose," "sloppy," or "undocumented," the level and sophistication of the new owner's policies and procedures need to be in keeping with the time and talents of the office staff and in keeping with sound small-business practices. No matter which policies and procedures are in place, the overhead of the newly acquired practice almost always seems to increase and has to be balanced with the value added by the new ownership interests. Finding the right balance between the expenses and policies of the new ownership and those of the former practice offers enlightened managers a real challenge if the practice is to be successful.

Support Services

Hospitals are uniquely positioned to bring a wide array of support services to the physician's practice. Smart management will examine carefully each service to gauge the potential for benefit and will avoid making across-the-board decisions to deploy the supporting cast of institutional players that might otherwise descend on the practice.

Measures of service, quality, and price can be used in determining the configuration of practice support services. Usually, the hospital is able to obtain superior price discounts in buying supplies, services, and equipment for the practice. However, even this apparent major advantage may be offset if the hospital's purchasing and supply distribution system is not responsive to the daily service and delivery needs of the practice.

Practice billing systems are virtually always based within the physician's office. However, management responsibility for billings, receivables, and collections may be based either within the practice or placed with the financial management of the hospital. Both plans have worked successfully. In the authors' experience, however, it is uncommon for an acute hospital's billing and accounts receivable priorities and know-how to mesh well with the vastly different characteristics of practice billing and receivables. Laboratory services (particularly referral lab), remote electrocardiograms, remote pulmonary function testing, and monitoring of radiographic equipment performance and maintenance are all natural extensions of the hospital when held to the same standards of service as independent vendors.

From the long list of hospital support services, the most critical is the role that can be played by the hospital's marketing professionals in enhancing and expanding the practice. Marketing can use sound principles of market research to identify changes in patterns, demographics, or referrals and can develop objective patient satisfaction surveys to focus on patient problems, new opportunities, and unmet needs. The use of a health care sales force and a physician liaison program can also develop new opportunities and help build new sources of patients and revenues. Marketing can develop brochures and newsletters and identify speaking opportunities for the physicians in order to gain increased visibility within the community.

Making Contract Terms Work

Making a success of practice management depends on the terms of the purchase agreement. How is the physician (or physician group) to be compensated? Is the physician an employee or independent contractor? Is physician compensation fixed, variable, or a combination of both? Are amounts received by the physician related to total fees charged or to cash collections? Is there a transitional period during which doctors practicing in the office have an assured level of income, or is the physician motivated to strive for peak productivity from the outset? How are accounts receivable and supply inventories treated under the agreement? Who pays for the physician's professional liability insurance?

Whatever the terms, you can be sure that physicians (as in all other businesses) respond to incentives embodied in the acquisition contract. The terms of the contract can contribute to successful practice management by creating practice incentives and a practice environment that motivate physicians and their employees to strive for the same goals sought by the acquiring institution. In short, mutually rewarding contract terms, such as terms that reward both the physicians and the health care system by achieving common objectives, require less management intervention and ensure higher levels of physician loyalty and productivity.

First-Year Escape Clauses

A clear-cut way to minimize the risk of a ruptured relationship in the early stages after the deal is closed is to establish a formal "engagement period" (or conditional purchase agreement) during the transition that allows either party to withdraw without penalty or hardship. One drawback of an engagement period is that it almost always postpones any major new capital investment by the buyer until both parties have signed on for a lasting marriage. However, a benefit is that it creates peak incentives for both parties to be on their best behavior while experiencing all the daily routines, trials, and, it is hoped, victories that will follow in the marriage itself.

Pitfalls at the Altar

Opportunities for misunderstandings at the altar of practice acquisition are seemingly infinite. Risks of a breakdown are especially high in an organization's earliest acquisitions. Here are six suggestions that will prevent management headaches and avoid unnecessary conflicts:

1. *Achieve a clear understanding of the acquired practice's decision-making process with participating physicians before moving ahead.* Allowing the decision-making roles between the physician, office manager, and organization buying the practice to remain unclear leads only to heartache and potential disaster. The physician knows his or her role will change but wants clear-cut guidelines and occasional reminders to modify long-established habits. This can be done by establishing a written list of the roles and responsibilities of both the physician and the practice manager. Some experienced practice buyers prefer to incorporate these delineated roles into the legal documents, while others prefer a more flexible format.

2. *Telegraph pay and benefits policies for practice employees in advance of the closing.* Even the earliest rumors of the practice's being acquired will set off speculation on salary increases and benefits improvements matched to hospital employment standards. Employees within the physician's office will inevitably seek answers and assurances from the physician that only the management of the acquiring organization can answer accurately.

   Many successful practice management organizations quickly learned that pay and benefit practices of the acute care hospital are simply too costly and out of sync with competitive practices in office settings. Telegraphing your organization's plans to hold pay and benefits at competitive levels is a real service to practice employees because it dispels unrealistic expectations. The timing of the initial communication to practice employees is critical. Astute physicians frequently include one or more practice employees in the early meetings with potential buyers. A straightforward explanation of how employees will be affected is appropriate immediately after agreement is reached on the terms of the purchase. Often this is weeks or months in advance of signing the actual legal agreements.

3. *Be crystal clear on how accounts receivable will be handled.* The language of business law, with all of its sophistication, still allows buyers and sellers to enjoy gross misunderstandings over how accounts receivable will be valued, collected, and paid to the seller. Be more astute than most in your first acquisition by including a well-written exhibit with your purchase agreement illustrating the mathematical treatment of receivables on the books at the time of closing.

4. *Spell out how practice-supply inventories will be valued.* Although routine business for public accounting firms, methods of valuing inventories purchased from the selling physician are new and unfamiliar territory for hospitals entering the practice acquisition game. Seek qualified advice in advance of negotiating the cash value of practice

inventories; spell out your agreement; and then verify that both parties share a common interpretation of the final contract language.

5. *If the office computer works, do not change it—yet!* Resist your natural corporate inclination to interject the hospital's information system into the acquired practice—unless your organization is among the few that enjoy a successful track record in computer networking with physician offices. But be sure to bring the testimonials of satisfied physician users to the negotiating table. Physicians skeptical of being tied to hospital information systems have ample reason without strong evidence to the contrary.

   Many physicians who have purchased their own office systems have strong attachments to "their system" and are genuinely fearful of losing that capability. Hospitals have a marginal record at best in bringing their hospital-oriented hardware and application software to the office practice environment. Lacking a compelling reason to do so, consider postponing a change in practice computer systems until after the transition is complete.

6. *Spell out professional compensation fee schedules, benefits, and physician and professional expenses.* Outlining terms of compensation, benefits, and responsibility for professional expenses verbally is both helpful and necessary but still falls short in ensuring a mutual understanding of the most sensitive subject of the negotiating process. Protect your organization's relationship by providing clearly drawn illustrations attached as exhibits to your acquisition agreement, and thoroughly discuss these delicate issues in detail well in advance of the contract signing.

Strengthening and Expanding the Practice

There are basically two methods for strengthening and expanding the physician's practice. The first is a strategy to retain as high a percentage of the existing patients as possible and the second is to develop new sources of patients. Retention strategies center around increasing the availability of the physician through more convenient and expanded hours (such as the evening hours and Saturday mornings) and strengthening the relationships between patients and physicians and/or office staff. Improved customer relations, follow-up phone calls, patient newsletters, and returning the patient and written reports promptly to the referring physician are all important strategies for increased patient satisfaction and practice growth.

Strategies directed to increasing patient volume include joining selected managed care plans that may bring a flow of new patients and joining one or more hospital-sponsored physician referral programs. Adding new clinical skills and new automated clinical office equipment should also enhance the practice and result in new patient populations. On-call coverage for the hospital emergency department or the urgent care center is another traditional method for increasing the flow of patients to the practice.

As the physician's most precious resource is his or her time and expertise, the availability to accept new patients and build long-term relationships cannot be overstated. Hospitals acquiring practices should always strive to increase both the efficiency of the physicians' time and the quality of the time spent with patients and referring physicians.

Ongoing Evaluation

Once purchased, management's evaluation of the practice's progress closely follows monitoring methods employed for other business acquisitions. Monthly reports on patient visits, gross charges, contract allowances, practice expenses, net income, cash collections, and accounts receivable are the fundamentals. Practice assessment surveys are also gaining widespread acceptance as a basic customer relations evaluation tool in practice management. These reports are generated by the practice manager and distributed to senior management, the physicians in the practice, and the office staff. It is imperative that the physicians, administration, and office staff meet on a monthly basis and carefully review these reports to ensure that the objectives and goals of the practice are being met.

Conclusion

The primary focus of an acquisition and enhancement strategy must be to keep the entrepreneurial spirit within the practice alive and growing. If the practice becomes too bureaucratic, there is a risk of losing both the financial incentives and the pride of ownership necessary for growth and competition. Only the hospital's real competitive strengths should be used in building the private practice. Experienced senior executives agree that to be successful the following guidelines should be considered:

- Make few and only necessary changes in the first few critical months.
- Involve the operating team and senior champion early in the negotiation process.
- Communicate effectively with the patients about changes.
- Integrate the practice carefully into the new health care family.
- Ensure that the financial incentives are clear and measurable.
- Ensure physician availability and convenient practice hours.

Although ambitious and somewhat risky, a physician acquisition and enhancement program can be one of the most successful strategies in meeting the challenges of today's competitive health care environment.

Index

and administrative support services for physician prac-
tices, 52–53
and clinical support services for
physician practices, 53–54
independent physician groups in,
55–57
influence of, on health maintenance organizations and
preferred provider organizations, 19
issue of control in, 67–68
and joint ventures, 63–67
motivations of, in accomplishing
product line and manpower
objectives, 21
Hospital visit, as aspect of practice
acquisition, 48–50

Imaging centers, 54
Independent physician groups,
assistance of, in practice
acquisition, 55–57, 120–22

Joint ventures, 10–11, 54
agreements for, 115
compensation, 119
medical directorships/consult-
ancies, 115–17
service site, 118–19
utilization of other practitioners, 117–18
formation of, between hospital
and physician practice,
63–67

Leased employees, treatment of,
under ERISA, 85
Legal issues, 71
antitrust laws, 85–86
charitable trust doctrine, 82
corporate practice acts and professional licensure require-
ments, 75–77
due diligence, 89–90

Employee Retirement Income
Security Act considerations,
82–85
liability and insurance, 88–89
Medicare/Medicaid fraud and
abuse prevention, 71–75
Medicare reimbursement, 86–88
tax considerations, 78–82
Letters of intent, in practice acquisition, 91–92
Liability insurance
as administrative support service,
53
as legal issue in practice acquisition, 89
Licensing, and practice acquisition,
77

Managed care program, joint risk
taking in, 54
Management fees, as fee splitting, 76
Manpower objectives, hospital motivations in accomplishing, 21
Market analysis, assessment of, in
evaluating practice, 97
Market share, role of hospitals in
protecting and expanding,
18–19
Medical director of hospital, as
member of practice acquisition team, 41
Medical directorships/consultancies,
54, 115
compensation in, 119
responsibilities of medical director
for, 115–17
service site for, 118–19
and utilization of other practitioners, 117–18
Medical society directories, identifying physicians for acquisition
in, 43–44
Medical staff, review of potential
acquisition candidates by,
45–46
Medicare/Medicaid fraud and abuse
prevention, as legal issue in
practice acquisition, 71–75